EMOTION REGULATION
IN CHILDREN AND ADOLESCENTS

EMOTION REGULATION IN CHILDREN AND ADOLESCENTS

A PRACTITIONER'S GUIDE

Michael A. Southam-Gerow

THE GUILFORD PRESS
New York   London

The author has checked with sources believed to be reliable in his effort to provide
information that is complete and generally in accord with the standards of practice that are
accepted at the time of publication. However, in view of the possibility of human error or
changes in behavioral, mental health, or medical sciences, neither the author, nor the editor
and publisher, nor any other party who has been involved in the preparation or publication
of this work warrants that the information contained herein is in every respect accurate or
complete, and they are not responsible for any errors or omissions or the results obtained from
the use of such information. Readers are encouraged to confirm the information contained in
this book with other sources.

Library of Congress Cataloging-in-Publication Data

Southam-Gerow, Michael A.
    Emotion regulation in children and adolescents : a practitioner's guide / by Michael A.
Southam-Gerow.
       p. cm.
    Includes bibliographical references and index.
    ISBN 978-1-4625-0829-7 (cloth : alk. paper)
    1. Emotions in children.   2. Emotions in adolescence.   3. Cognitive therapy for
children.   4. Cognitive therapy for teenagers.   I. Title.
    BF723.E6S68 2013
    155.4′124—dc23
                                                                2012036624

About the Author

Michael A. Southam-Gerow, PhD, is Associate Professor in the Departments of Psychology and Pediatrics at Virginia Commonwealth University (VCU), Co-director of the Anxiety Clinic at VCU's Monroe Park Campus, and Director of Graduate Studies for VCU's Department of Psychology. He is also Director of Quality and Performance at PracticeWise, LLC, a private company offering therapists and agencies training in evidence-based approaches to children's mental health care. Dr. Southam-Gerow's research focuses on the dissemination and implementation of evidence-based treatments (EBTs) for mental health problems in children and adolescents. He completed a project funded by the National Institute of Mental Health (NIMH) that adapts EBTs for anxiety and depression in a large public community mental health clinic in central Virginia through the application of a partnership model. He also studies treatment integrity, including therapist adherence to and competence in delivering specific treatment models, and is Co-Principal Investigator with Dr. Bryce McLeod on a 5-year grant from NIMH to develop treatment integrity measures. Dr. Southam-Gerow's other research interests include the study of emotion processes such as emotion regulation and emotion understanding in children and adolescents and how these processes relate to child psychopathology and the provision of mental health care in pediatric primary care settings. An Associate Editor of the *Journal of Clinical Child and Adolescent Psychology*, Dr. Southam-Gerow is the author of dozens of scholarly papers and is on multiple journal review boards.

Acknowledgments

On the face of it, writing a book is a crazy endeavor. Hours spent in solitude. Missed deadlines that create gut-wrenching anxiety. A project full of fits and starts, seemingly endless. What made writing this particular book worth all the effort is that its topic, emotion-related treatment interventions for children and adolescents, is both critically important for the field of mental health treatment and one about which I am passionate. For more than a dozen years I have believed that someone should write a book on this topic. When given the opportunity, I jumped at the chance.

Although most of the glory for writing a book goes to the author on the cover, many individuals who do not appear on the cover contribute to the final project. I am indebted and grateful to a number of people who have contributed in one way or another to this book. Among them are my academic and intellectual mentors, who have helped me develop as a scientist and a writer, including my high school English teacher, Mrs. Kircher; my undergraduate writing mentors Bert Hornback, Charles Bambach, and Tish Ezekiel; my graduate school professors Phil Kendall, Jay Efran, Rick Heimberg, Larry Steinberg, Bill Overton, and Rob Fauber; my graduate school friends in the Child and Adolescent Anxiety Disorders Clinic at Temple University, who taught me all I know about therapy with kids, Serena Ashmore-Callahan, Erika Brady, Tamar Chansky, Brian Chu, Ellen Flannery-Schroeder, Elizabeth Gosch (who first taught me how to do cognitive-behavioral therapy for anxiety), Aude Henin, Martha Kane, Amy Krain, Abbe Marrs-Garcia, Suzie Panichelli-Mindel, and Melissa Warman; my current colleagues and collaborators Robert Allin, Marc Atkins, Doug Bilski, Eric Daleiden, Al Haskell, Ann Garland, Kimberly Hoagwood, Aaron Hogue, Yo Jackson, Michele MacPhee, Bryce McLeod, Mary Katherine O'Connor, Sonja Schoenwald, Scott Vrana, John Weisz, and Janice Zeman; my tireless graduate students at Virginia Commonwealth University (VCU), including Alyssa Ward, Kim Goodman, Ruth Brown, and Shannon Hourigan (all

PhDs now), and Alexis Quinoy, Cassidy Arnold, Carrie Bair, Adriana Rodriguez, and Julia Cox (all working on their doctorates). I am also grateful to the dozens of therapists (too numerous to mention) whom I have supervised at the Anxiety Clinic at VCU, and the hundreds of therapists I have trained in California, Hawaii, Maine, Massachusetts, Minnesota, Washington, D.C., and Virginia whose work has inspired and taught me so much about therapy with children and adolescents.

Two of my professional colleagues warrant special mention. First, Phil Kendall, my graduate school advisor, to whom I am especially grateful for having seen something in the raw talent I was when I arrived at Temple University in the early 1990s. He taught me not only how to do cognitive-behavioral therapy but also how to be an academic researcher. Thanks, Phil! And thanks, too, to Bruce Chorpita, who served as a role model for me as I navigated the early stages of my career and with whom I developed a productive and enjoyable collaboration. I am glad we had lunch that day in Boston!

I also thank Anne Marie Albano, who encouraged me to write this book. Her support has been most appreciated. Thanks, too, to The Guilford Press, especially Kitty Moore, Senior Editor, and Alice Broussard, Senior Assistant Editor, for their support during the process. Alice, in particular, deserves a badge of honor for her excellent editorial suggestions throughout the process. She always had kind words for my drafts while also delivering keen and probing feedback.

I have been fortunate enough to receive financial support from the National Institute of Mental Health and VCU for research that contributed to the ideas expressed in this book. I am particularly grateful to current and former program officers at NIMH Joel Sherrill, Serene Olin, and Heather Ringeisen, whose encouragement early in my career was pivotal.

On a more personal level, I am incredibly appreciative of the support from my family. My parents, Bob and Carolyn, nurtured in me an insatiable hunger for knowledge and a passion for hard work, both of which were important in the process of writing this book. My children, Zen and Evelyn, have been an ever-giving source of love and encouragement, and they have been glad to remind me of the need for modesty when I think I know all there is to know about parenting and childhood. Finally, I thank my wife, Kim, whose support and belief in me is as precious a gift as any given me. I can still hear that harp playing in Seattle.

Contents

PART I

BACKGROUND ON EMOTIONS AND EMOTION REGULATION

CHAPTER 1

Introduction

THE IMPORTANCE
OF EMOTION-RELATED INTERVENTIONS

Treatment developers have long neglected the topic of emotion, particularly since the rise to prominence of behavior and cognitive-behavioral therapy (CBT). The neglect of emotion is somewhat surprising, given the prominence of emotion in the CBT model. The basic CBT model includes three variables, often depicted as circles arranged in a triangle with double-headed arrows connecting each to each: (1) actions, (2) thoughts, and (3) feelings. The idea is simple: What one does influences what one thinks and how one feels. And how one feels influences what ones does and what one thinks. And so on. The model makes no predictions about where the cycle starts or where it will end. Instead, it simply summarizes the idea that thoughts, feelings, and actions are related to and influence one another.

Although emotion is depicted in the model, most CBT approaches emphasize interventions aimed at behavior or cognition. One reason has been that the science of emotion has lagged behind the science of behavior and cognition, although certainly not for lack of interest. Scientists and philosophers have been fascinated by emotion for centuries. Early Greek philosophers opined on emotions and so-called "passions." Aristotle, one of the earliest documented thinkers to expound on the topic, may be one of the first to articulate the connection among emotions, thoughts, and actions. Philosophers and artists through the ages have written about emotions. Some portrayed emotions as "passions" that weakened humans could succumb to or overcome by using the rational mind. Others offered a more positive view of emotions, noting their importance in interpersonal interactions and their utility in helping us better understand what is important to us.

More recently, scientists like Charles Darwin and William James theorized about and studied emotion and its role in human life. However, particularly within

3

psychology, behavioral and cognitive sciences received a lot of attention in the middle and later years of the 20th century, especially with regard to the development of treatments for mental health problems. A review of randomized controlled trials published from the 1980s to the early 2000s will attest to the prominence of behavioral and cognitive-behavioral treatments, based in part on the findings from basic behavioral and cognitive science.

However, beginning in the late 1980s and continuing through the 1990s and 2000s, a renewed interest in emotion science swept the field of human behavior. Although there were several contributing factors to the focus on emotion, a primary reason has been the advances in neuroscience. As the field began to better understand emotional circuitry in the brain, emotion became "observable" in a sense and thus was viewed as a legitimate focus for science. Furthermore, as evidence accumulated on the effects of various treatments, including CBT, treatment developers and therapists alike began to identify areas for improvement, based in part on the fact that, as good as the treatments were, many clients were still not improving as much as they deemed possible.

Partly as a result of these occurrences, interest in integrating emotion into a variety of treatment models burgeoned. In child and adolescent therapy alone, there have been numerous examples of prevention and treatment interventions targeting emotional development. One example is Promoting Alternative Thinking Strategies (PATHS), a prevention program that helps school-age children develop emotional competence (Greenberg, Kusche, Cook, & Quamma, 1995). PATHS includes interventions designed specifically to influence social and neurological development related to emotion. For instance, the program attempts to target frontal lobe involvement in emotional development by teaching self-control strategies such as self-talk, thereby promoting what is called vertical control (i.e., higher-order processing, emotion regulation by frontal lobes). The PATHS program also focuses on emotion education concepts such as labeling and identifying emotions, promoting what is called horizontal communication (i.e., information processing that occurs across the two halves of the neocortex, or, more simply, better right brain–left brain communication; Greenberg & Kusche, 2002).

In addition, other scientists have developed and tested emotion-infused treatments for youths with diagnosable psychopathology. For example, Cindy Suveg and her colleagues (Suveg, Kendall, Comer, & Rabin, 2006) introduced a program called emotion-focused cognitive-behavioral treatment (ECBT), which focuses on children with anxiety disorders. The program includes many interventions found in CBT for anxiety, including psychoeducation on anxiety, cognitive skills, problem-solving skills, exposure, plus content that specifically addresses emotion understanding and emotion regulation skills. Another recent emotion-infused treatment developed and tested by Maria Kovacs and her collagues (Kovacs et al., 2006) is called contextual emotion-regulation therapy (CERT). CERT emphasizes emotion regulation in an interpersonal context, with a focus on identifying maladaptive responses to dysphoria and reducing the impact of contextual factors that might maintain the responses.

In the program, youths learn a variety of skills, including information about emotional development and emotion recognition skills. Both of these treatments have garnered preliminary empirical support.

Interest in emotion theory and research applied to treatment of adults is arguably even "hotter." Among the first to emphasize emotion was Marsha Linehan (1993) in her development of dialectical behavior therapy (DBT). The emotional aspects of DBT include an emphasis on "acceptance" strategies with regard to emotional experiences. The acceptance and commitment therapy (ACT) model developed by Steve Hayes and colleagues (Hayes, Strosahl, & Wilson, 1999) is another approach incorporating similar ideas—that one way to help clients with psychological distress lies in helping them accept their emotional experiences. Many other treatments that integrate emotion-related interventions have been developed and tested for adults (see Mennin & Farach, 2007, for review), a discussion of which would take this brief introduction too far afield.

Clearly, then, interest in emotion-related interventions for children and adolescents (and adults) is a hot topic. However, as I was pitching about for a dissertation topic in the mid-1990s, few if any of these programs existed. As a result, I drew on my own clinical experiences to date as a young CBT therapist and recognized that emotion was "missing" from the model. Specifically, children with mental health problems had emotion-related gaps in their understanding that might not be adequately treated by a focus on behaviors and thoughts. The research stemming from my observations suggested that children with anxiety problems, for example, were indeed struggling to understand emotions; in fact, children without such problems were also struggling to understand emotions (Southam-Gerow & Kendall, 2000). We now have more than a decade's worth of studies from multiple investigators that support this idea (see Suveg, Southam-Gerow, Goodman, & Kendall, 2007).

My other research interest concerns the adaptation of treatments for use in new contexts. Of particular interest is taking treatments with an evidence base from research studies and working with therapists in other settings to adapt those treatments for the clients they see. While conducting such a study in central Virginia with therapists in a public mental health clinic, I received feedback through informal and formal (e.g., focus groups) means suggesting that evidence-based treatments needed more focus on emotion (see Southam-Gerow, Hourigan, & Allin, 2009). As part of a study we were doing, I received additional feedback from therapists on this point and wrote a set of treatment modules on emotion that served as a basis for this book. The modules found herein were written and used in our study working with youths and families in a public mental health clinic.

SCOPE OF THE BOOK

First, and perhaps most important, this book is *not* designed as a stand-alone treatment program. Rather, the treatment strategies described in this book are designed to be modular, a concept described in more detail in Chapter 5. One characteristic of modular approaches is that they can be "plugged in" to other approaches, like new Lego pieces that can be attached to an existing structure or model. In short, this book contains several sets of treatment interventions that can be used singly or in combination and with other interventions.

Which Problem Areas?

The strategies in this book are designed for children or adolescents who have any of several emotion-related deficits, including poor emotional awareness, limited emotional understanding, poorly developed empathy skills, or poor emotion regulation. Given that these emotion-related problems exist in a wide variety of clients presenting for mental health treatment, the strategies in this book are not designed for a specific set of child problems or a specific DSM disorder. This fact distinguishes the book from many others, which tend to be designed for a specific diagnostic group or specific problem area. Instead, this book is designed to help youths with many different types of problems and who, as part of their struggles, are lacking in some emotional competencies. For example, a young child with anxiety problems and an adolescent with severe conduct problems may share a lack of emotion understanding, and this book is designed to help both of them.

In fact, the strategies are designed to apply to children with a variety of DSM diagnoses. Aside from the most common problems encountered in most outpatient settings (e.g., mild to moderate behavior problems, anxiety and depressive disorders), it is possible to use some of the interventions with children with Asperger syndrome, although a specialty text should be used in conjunction (e.g., White, 2011). Of course, to follow Gordon Paul's (1967) adage carefully, it should be clearly stated for whom the strategies may have limited applicability. The problems for which these interventions may be less germane, at least as a primary focus of treatment, would include: psychotic disorders, mental retardation, and moderate to severe autism. In addition, although the modules here may help children with severe forms of conduct disorder or youth with chronic suicidal behavior, they may not be well suited as a primary focus for such clients, especially given the fact that there are currently well-designed and tested treatments for these problems.

Which Age Groups?

The interventions described in the book are designed for children of elementary school age or older. Examples in the book will be tailored to differing age groups to demonstrate how to use the interventions across the developmental span. Thus the book was written for therapy practiced with children and adolescents. However, some therapists may find the strategies useful with their adult cases, with some modifications. In short, the interventions apply across a broad developmental range but interventions should be adapted on the basis of the youth's age or maturity.

Which Settings?

Another consideration for using the interventions in the book is the settings in which they apply. Most treatments in the evidence base to date have been tested in outpatient or school settings. Hence, because the interventions described are derived or inspired in part by many of these evidence-based treatment programs, those settings are certainly appropriate. However, having consulted with therapists in the use of these and similar strategies in many other settings (e.g., residential, day treatment, home-based), I have found that their use in other settings has been useful.

STRUCTURE OF THE BOOK

The book is organized into two parts. Part I provides the conceptual framework for the treatment modules contained in Part II. In Chapter 2, I provide background on the many emotion-related constructs discussed in the book. This chapter is designed to provide a general background, enough to help the reader understand and apply the modules described in the second part of the book. Interested readers are referred to other sources for more in-depth examination of the complex empirical and theoretical issues involved in emotion science. Chapter 3 provides a very brief overview of the importance of assessment and describes specific tools to measure emotion-related constructs. In Chapter 4, functional analysis is introduced as a specific assessment procedure designed to facilitate treatment planning. This chapter warrants some justification. Why include such a chapter in this book? As mentioned, one of my primary research interests concerns the adaptation of evidence-based treatments through partnerships with clinicians in diverse settings. That work has led to my understanding that treatment conceptualization is central for teaching and applying specific treatment strategies. In central Virginia, we have successfully used functional analysis as a means of flexibly applying evidence-based modular treatment strategies to complex, multiproblem cases. Thus, because functional analysis was an important part of how the modules contained in the book were developed and applied, the reader will need to understand functional analysis. Chapter 5 describes how to translate functional analysis into a treatment plan. Because the treatment strategies described in the book are in modular form, I review the concept of modularity. Modularity is a popular idea now in the field of mental health treatment. However, the term is used to refer to a number of different approaches to treatment, not all of which are truly modular. Thus Chapter 5 defines modularity and describes why it is important in applying the strategies that comprise the bulk of the book. Chapter 5 also provides a clear description of how modularity and functional analysis work together in delivering the modules in the book. The final chapter of the first part of the book, Chapter 6, describes how to involve caregivers in treatment, how to use the modules with diverse populations, and how to engage difficult clients.

The second part of the book includes eight modules— (1) Emotion Awareness Skills, (2) Emotion Understanding Skills, (3) Empathy Skills, (4) Emotion Regulation Skills I: Prevention Skills, (5) Emotion Regulation Skills II: Mastery, (6) Emotion Regulation Skills III: Expression Skills, (7) Emotion Regulation Skills IV: Basic Cognitive Skills, and (8) Emotion Regulation Skills V: Emotion-Specific Cognitive Skills—describing eight different treatment strategies. The modules are ordered in a typical developmental sequence. As noted in Chapter 5, though, ordering in modularity is not set in stone. Thus one could use all eight modules in the book with several cases but do them in a different order each time.

CONCLUSION

An important aspect of helping children and adolescents with mental health problems lies in helping them learn about and sort through their emotional experiences by focusing on the emotions. Through the modules in this book, a therapist can build a treatment plan that will help ameliorate the emotional development deficits of a wide variety of clients. This book offers ideas for ways to help clients recognize and respond to emotion cues in themselves and others; strategies for helping clients understand how emotions "work" and what they might mean; and a variety of techniques to help clients learn how to manage the sometimes confusing array of emotional experiences they encounter and struggle with in their daily lives.

CHAPTER 2

Conceptual Background
The Science of Emotions

Behaviorism, a guiding theoretical perspective in psychology for many years, has generated important findings on the determinants of human behavior. Insights gleaned from classical conditioning, operant conditioning, and social learning paradigms have contributed both scientifically and practically to our understanding of human development and mental health problems. Few question the importance of behavioral theory in moving the field of psychological treatments forward; however, in eschewing internal variables, behaviorism may have left out important mental factors from the equation. When researchers and therapists sought to bring meaning-making back under scientific scrutiny, that effort was called the "cognitive revolution." The impact of cognitive theory and research was considerable, and integration of the cognitive and behavioral perspectives emerged as a fruitful one (although not without its detractors). Most in the field are now aware of the strong evidence base underlying cognitive-behavioral treatments for a wide variety of psychological problems.

Despite its many strengths, the emphasis on cognitive and behavioral factors may have led researchers and clinicians to undervalue the role of emotion in clinical practice. Although the field commonly refers to "emotional disorders" or "emotional problems," and emotion is considered a cornerstone of human experience, until recently, many theoretical models had not adequately considered the role of emotion in development and psychopathology. Fortunately, research efforts by a diverse group of investigators suggest that the field has been experiencing an "emotion revolution." Research in developmental psychopathology has led to increased emphasis on the importance of emotional processes in normative and atypical development.

In addition, advances in neuroscience and psychophysiology have greatly expanded our knowledge about the neural and other psychophysiological concomitants of emotion and how these might influence adjustment. Furthermore, an interest in emotion has been fueled by the concepts of emotional intelligence, emotional competence, and emotional education that have burgeoned in educational, scientific, medical, and legislative domains. Finally, and most germane to this book, concepts and findings from emotion science have influenced the development and adaptation of conceptual and treatment models for a wide variety of psychological problems (e.g., Greenberg, 2002; Mennin & Farach, 2007; Suveg et al., 2007).

This book offers practical treatment techniques based on findings from emotion science. Before describing those techniques, some background on several central concepts will be helpful. The present chapter provides a primer on key ideas that will be used throughout the book, including *emotion, emotional competence, emotion awareness, emotion understanding, empathy, emotion regulation,* and *emotion socialization.* The following discussion is meant to be illustrative rather than exhaustive. Each of these concepts could be the focus of an entire book (and often are). Here, the goal is to provide a broad overview as a way to get a foothold in the fast-growing area of emotion science.

EMOTION

Questions about the nature of human emotion have engendered a long and unsettled—although productive—debate throughout history among diverse disciplines. Within psychology, there have been considerable differences in recent theoretical positions on emotion, and to discuss them all is a topic for another book. For practical reasons, only a few of the primary positions taken by emotion theorists are discussed. The interested reader is referred to several other resources for more depth and breadth on this topic (e.g., Ekman, 1992; Frijda, 1986; Izard, Kagan, & Zajonc, 1984; Lewis, Haviland-Jones, & Barrett, 2008).

> **emotion:** the affective aspects of human experience; emotion involves a complex interaction of biological, psychological, and environmental influences.

Working definitions of emotion have evolved from considerations of the structure of emotion to the function of emotion as adaptive and motivational (Campos, Campos, & Barrett, 1989; Campos, Frankel, & Camras, 2004; Izard et al., 1984; Saarni, 1999). Early approaches focused on the biological bases of emotion, including the focus of Charles Darwin on the bioevolutionary origins of emotion and the work of William James, whose thoughts on the matter have been pithily summarized as, "I am afraid of the bear because I run from the bear." These early approaches noted the close association between often intense physiological experiences and the "feeling" of an emotion.

Theorists following in a physiological and structural tradition have focused on several topics, including (1) which emotions may be basic ones (and thus perhaps "hardwired" into humans via evolution); (2) how emotions are displayed in the face and body; (3) how emotions are "experienced" in the brain, with particular emphasis on which brain areas may be involved in which emotions; and (4) the universality (or not) of emotions across cultures. It is not accurate to say that biological and structural approaches to emotion differ radically from the more psychological approaches that follow. Indeed, theorists on both sides often agree on the fundamentals. However, for the purposes of this overview, it is useful to note that some theories emphasize the biology of emotion and others emphasize what we may call the psychology of emotion.

The psychological theories, most of which can be described as "functionalist," often emphasize the importance of appraisal in emotion. The emphasis on appraisal arose in the middle of the last century and was a reaction, like the cognitive revolution, to what was perceived as a lack of emphasis on the relevance of meaning to emotional experience, particularly meaning in a social context. So, for example, Joseph Campos, a major figure among functionalists, defined emotions as "processes of establishing, maintaining, or disrupting the relations between the person and the internal or external environment" on matters important to the individual (Campos et al., 1989, p. 395). In other words, emotions motivate a person to adapt to the environment and to modify the environment to fit his or her goals/concerns (cf. Frijda, 1986). Similarly, Arnold defined emotion thusly: "Emotion is the felt tendency toward an object judged suitable, or away from an object judged unsuitable, reinforced by specific bodily changes according to the type of emotion" (Arnold & Gasson, 1954, p. 294).

The functionalist conceptualization is closely aligned with a psychoevolutionary view: emotions have evolved to organize physiological systems (the biological and psychoevolutionary component) and to facilitate an adaptive response to important events (the functionalist component—see, e.g., Darwin, 1872; Ekman, 1992; Gray, 1990; Izard et al., 1984). For example, Izard's (1977) differential emotions theory suggests that emotion is associated with a unique action tendency or behavioral response pattern. An action tendency can effectively short-circuit more laborious cognitive processes (reason, problem solving) to efficiently organize behavior in the face of danger (cf. Gray, 1990).

Although many theorists take a functionalist view on emotion, their emphases differ. For example, some have emphasized relational aspects of emotion, such that the interpersonal meaning of events becomes central to defining and understanding emotions (e.g., Lazarus, 1991). Similarly, social constructivist perspectives emphasize relational meaning, although these theories note the active role that the individual takes in ascribing emotional meaning to events, especially when considering the so-called self-referential emotions such as shame and embarrassment (e.g., Lewis, 2008; cf. Frijda, 1986).

In short, although theory on emotion has a long history and is often diverse, most current accounts of emotion focus on biological and evolutionary underpinnings of emotion—that is, that emotion serves a critical role in human survival. Furthermore, most accounts emphasize functional aspects of emotion, particularly with regard to the function(s) emotion serves in interpersonal relationships: emotion tells us what (and who) is important to us and motivates us to maintain or disrupt our relations with people and objects.

With the definition of emotion explored, the next section focuses on multiple emotion-related constructs, beginning with *emotional competence.*

EMOTIONAL COMPETENCE

Emotional competence is, in a sense, a primary goal of emotional development. Considerable research suggests that emotional competence (or social-emotional competence, as it is sometimes called) is related to numerous outcomes including mental/behavioral health, academic success, and social adaptation (Masten, Burt, & Coatsworth, 2006; Saarni, 1999). But what exactly is emotional competence? Like emotion, there is no single accepted definition of emotional competence, despite its acknowledged importance. The science of emotion is so relatively young that there are few givens, and much of the conceptual territory remains in open dispute, awaiting further evidence.

> **emotional competence:** the ability of an individual to function adaptively in many contexts across many different aspects of emotional functioning.

Saarni (1999) has outlined a broad and comprehensive definition of emotional competence that is widely cited (e.g., Denham, 2006; Trentacosta & Izard, 2007). She identifies contributors to emotional competence, such as the person's learning history and sense of morality and several components relevant to the development of emotional competence. Several of Saarni's components of emotional competence are listed in Table 2.1. Each of these skills warrants brief discussion.

TABLE 2.1. Select Component Constructs Related to Emotional Competence

• Emotion awareness of self and others	• Emotion regulation
• Emotion understanding	• Emotion socialization
• Empathy/sympathy	

Emotion Awareness

Emotion awareness is thought to be one of the most basic skills relevant to emotional competence, and it involves introspection into one's own and others' emotional experience (e.g., Stegge & Terwogt, 2007). Saarni (1999) distinguishes awareness of one's own emotions from awareness of others' emotions. Emotion awareness and emotion understanding, a topic discussed shortly, are interrelated. In this book, effort is made to keep the concepts distinct, but as the reader will see, the distinction is somewhat artificial. Understanding emotions—both abstractly and in the context of one's own direct experiences—clearly affects emotion awareness. In the same way, emotional experiences (i.e., lived experience that involves emotion—much of life!) that increase emotion awareness affect emotion understanding.

> **emotion awareness:** knowing about one's own (or others') emotional experience.

Considering emotion awareness of one's own emotions, Saarni notes that a prerequisite is a sense of self. That is, one must recognize that one exists separately from others as a (largely) coherent self who can be aware of emotions. With this as the starting point, emotional awareness then stems from noticing and analyzing a variety of physiological, cognitive, and social cues that lead one to identify one's own emotional state. There are several aspects of that state to notice, and awareness of them does not develop in absolute synchrony.

First, emotions involve physiological changes throughout the body. Indeed, learning the meanings of these changes is a critical developmental task. The science of emotion is perhaps most advanced in this arena insofar as a number of physiological and particularly brain systems related to specific emotions have been identified. Although there is not a perfect one-to-one correspondence between these physiological events and the "experience" of a particular emotion, one may learn that the pattern of "flushed face, racing heart, fists clenching, 'seeing' red" represents the body's feelings associated with anger. Furthermore, one can learn to tell the difference between an uncomfortable feeling in one's stomach due to anxiety and similar feelings resulting from bad chili.

Second, awareness of emotions involves not only knowing that feelings involve complex physiological responses in the body, but also involves awareness of several characteristics of emotions. First, feelings vary in intensity and duration. That is, children learn that feelings can be "big" or "small" and that they can last a long time or disappear quickly. In addition, children become aware that feelings do not occur in a linear, one-at-a-time fashion. Instead, more than one feeling occurs at the same time, as when a child feels anxious during her soccer game because the ball is coming her way, excited at the prospect of kicking the ball hard, and happy to see a loved one on the sidelines. These characteristics of emotion reflect various aspects of how feelings work, as is explored later in the discussion of emotion understanding.

Finally, emotions are contextual: they occur in relationship to something or someone. Emotions are thus affected by the actions of others, events occurring in the world, and the "events" in one's own inner life. Let's take a simple example. Imagine a child whose sister has just grabbed his toy and is running away from him, laughing. The child begins to experience a variety of physiological experiences: his face flushes, his fists clench, his eyes narrow. These responses constitute the first step just discussed (the flood of bodily feelings). Imagine that the child places high value on this toy. It is his *prized* toy! He may also recall that this is not the first time this week that his sister has snatched one of his possessions. Furthermore, imagine that his mom is out of the room and she has, in the last few days, seemed to take his sister's side more often than his. Finally, it is late in the day; he is tired and getting hungry. All of this information is relevant to the child's experience and awareness of feelings he might be experiencing, like anger.

These contextual cues are most often and most easily recognized post hoc. That is, it is much easier for the child to understand later that he was angry because of the past slights, the high value placed on the toy, and the late hour of his supper. Therapists, on the other hand, often immediately see the benefits of using the context cues both in the moment as well as in a preventive way. Indeed, if a child can be coached to become aware in the moment that this sort of situation with his sister is one where he gets really angry, he may be able to marshal some regulatory forces and avoid an ugly scene. For example, he can tell himself, "She is just trying to get my goat. I don't have to let her annoy me. I will get my toy back." As prevention, his awareness of the types of situations that make him particularly (and "dangerously") angry, helps him take steps to reduce the chances for anger, or at least take steps to reduce its impact. In short, awareness of contextual cues can be powerful allies in efforts to engage in adaptive emotion regulation.

The developmental process of awareness of other's emotions is similar in some respects, although there is understandably greater reliance on observable cues. For example, facial expressions and bodily cues represent clear (but not completely reliable) signals of others' emotional states. In addition, awareness involves calculus of the contextual factors, including whether a given situation is likely to create anger, sadness, or joy in the other person. The discerning reader knows that outward expression and the specifics of the situation alone are incomplete guides to the emotions of others. Indeed, understanding that emotion is an "inner state" and that others can mask that inner state is important knowledge that a child must possess so that she can develop a strong and accurate awareness of others' emotions.

Complex as the calculus of contextual factors is for gauging one's own emotions, it is even more so when determining the emotions of others because one has to place oneself in the position of the other person (i.e., use perspective taking) and imagine how the situation would make that particular person feel. Knowing a person well can serve as an important guide in assessing his or her emotional state. For example, imagine that a child sees another child about to receive an award at a swim meet. It will help the observing child to determine the recipient's emotions if he knows any of the following possible facts about the recipient: (1) she lied about accomplishments to receive the award; (2) she has never received an award before and this represents a major accomplishment in her life; (3) she has received this award several times in the past and no one else wants or merits the award on her team; or (4) she does not like others paying attention to her, whether for good or bad actions. Knowing those facts, the observer can make a reasonable assessment of the recipient's action. Without such knowledge, chances are slimmer.

In summary, emotion awareness is a key component of emotional competence. Recognizing body cues, identifying aspects of the experience of emotion, and learning the many contextual factors associated with emotion pave the way for adaptive self-regulation and for adaptive interaction with others in our social world. Module 1 focuses on the development of emotion awareness skills.

Emotion Understanding

Emotion understanding refers to conscious knowledge about emotion processes (e.g., emotion states, emotion regulation) or beliefs about how emotions work (cf. attribution system of Izard & Harris, 1995). In a sense, emotion understanding encompasses knowledge from emotional awareness as well as knowledge about the concepts that follow—particularly emotion regulation. Thus emotion understanding may be thought of as the cornerstone of emotional competence building as it interacts with the other components of emotional competence.

> **emotion understanding:** conscious knowledge about emotion processes (e.g., emotion states, emotion regulation) or beliefs about how emotions work.

Given the fact that emotion understanding is such a broad and important construct, relatively more space is dedicated to it here. The discussion takes a developmental perspective, starting with basic emotion knowledge and moving toward the more complex. Emotion understanding includes (1) recognition of emotion expression (i.e., facial, bodily); (2) knowledge about the causes of and cues for one's own (and others') emotions; (3) an understanding of multiple emotions; (4) knowledge about the methods of intentionally using emotion expression to communicate to others (or vice versa; e.g., display rules, hiding emotions); and (5) knowledge about the methods of coping with emotions (i.e., emotion regulation). Regarding this last item, a discussion of emotion regulation occurs later in the chapter. Here, the discussion is on *knowing* about emotion regulation (i.e., knowing one can change one's emotions), not *doing* emotion regulation.

Recognition of Emotion Expression

Children recognize facial expressions associated with emotions at an early age—at least by the age of 2 years—and some investigators have suggested that infants as young as 10 weeks evidence some form of comprehension of emotion from facial expressions (Izard & Harris, 1995). However, some question remains as to whether these early reactions represent recognition of emotion in another, recognition of a signal with ramifications for self, or simple mimesis. Regardless, by age 2, most children are using emotion labels for facial expressions and are talking about emotion topics (e.g., Camras & Allison, 1985). Furthermore, their ability to discriminate facial expressions shows a developmental progression, with negative emotions (e.g., sadness, anger) proving more difficult. In addition, older children are better able to select appropriate facial expressions for people in situations involving emotional arousal.

Causes and Cues of Emotions

Regarding the causes (and effects) of emotion and the cues used in inferring emotion, developmental research has detailed a progression from situation-bound, "behavioral" explanations of emotion to broader, more mentalistic understandings. In other words, a child's early understanding of emotion is based on her theory that the world causes her feelings: "I am mad because someone broke the toy." As she develops, her explanations of emotions move inward, focusing on internal causes: "I am mad because that broken toy was important to me," or, "I am mad because I thought the person who broke my toy was my friend."

The transition away from behavioral theories of emotion toward the internal theories is not absolute, of course. The child's understanding of the causes of emotions becomes more nuanced as she develops. She learns to identify the many determinants of a particular emotion, including current information and historical factors. For instance, she can learn that the anger she experienced when her toy was broken was linked not only to the simple fact that her sister broke the toy. It is also linked to (1) how much she enjoys the toy presently, (2) the fact that the toy was given to her by a grandfather who is now dead, and (3) her own feelings of guilt over having broken her sister's toy last year. It is also worth noting that research indicates even young children can understand some limited "mentalistic" conceptions of emotions such as, "I am mad because I liked the toy." But is only with development (and adequate experience) that children develop the nuanced view of emotion that indicates a high level of emotional competence.

As children develop, their emotional inferences evolve to contain more complex and differentiated uses of several types of information. For example, children learn to use historical facts and personal information, such as when a child can know that a friend is afraid of water and does not swim, and so a pool party will make that friend anxious. Children also learn about what is referred to as display rules. These are unwritten social customs about how and when one may display certain emotions. The classic example involves reciept of an unwanted gift. In this situation, a child receives a "bad" gift, like a pair of old, unappealing socks. If the child is alone, it is acceptable for him to display his feelings of disappointment. However, if the gift giver is present, he must display a different feeling—gratitude. Development also influences emotional inferencing. When children are younger, things their parents do are important to their feelings; as a teen, things their peers do are often more salient for their emotions. Another factor children must learn about emotions is that goals or beliefs are influential. For example, assume Michelle and her friend Taya are playing a game of soccer. Their team is losing, a disappointing situation on its face. Assume, though, Taya knows that Michelle is more excited about going to her friend Alyssa's house after the game than she is about the game itself. As a result, Taya knows that Michelle won't be very disappointed if their team loses.

An understanding of the effects of emotion is also a developmental achievement for children. One emotion can temporally color subsequent emotions or events. For example, a child who has had a bad bus ride home from school may react with more anger or annoyance than usual when asked to do homework upon arriving home. Such emotional effects often persist beyond the immediate or "triggering" event, although they typically wane over time. With development, understanding of these phenomena becomes more systematic, discriminating, and integrative, with valence (positive or negative) and target of the emotion having moderating influences on this development. For example, if a child really wanted to go out with his friends, he would time his request with his parents so that either he asked right after he had done a good job on a school project or chore, or he asked long after he had made a mistake (like forgetting to feed the dog).

Multiple Emotions

Children also develop an understanding that they (and others) experience more than one emotion at the same time. This understanding is not only that emotions can (and often do) occur simultaneously, but also that emotions can be directed toward more than one target. This sort of understanding is directly related to ambivalent feelings, such as when a child realizes that she can be both angry at and still loving toward her parents. This understanding is not innate; research suggests that most preschool children, even when trained to identify all of the relevant information, deny that feelings can occur simultaneously. Development of the understanding of multiple emotions involves adding complexity to the simple idea of having more than one feeling simultaneously. A child must learn that these two feelings can (1) be differently valenced (e.g., happy and angry vs. happy and proud); (2) be of varying intensities (e.g., really happy and a little angry vs. really happy and really proud); and (3) involve different targets (e.g., happy about his birthday cake but angry that his sister blew out the candles). Understanding multiple emotions is aided greatly by understanding that internal factors like beliefs and goals can "cause" emotions.

Intentional Use of Emotions to Communicate

There is perhaps no more important development in emotion understanding than the insight that one can hide and change one's feelings. The understanding is important because, as the rest of this book details, learning to change how we feel is crucial to social adaptation. Hiding and changing emotions are obviously different things, but they both have as a key component the notion that emotions are malleable. In the case of hiding, one learns that one can feel something and yet not let anyone, or only let select people, know. In fact, a child can actually show people that he feels one thing when inside he feels another.

When a child understands that he can change his emotions, he is essentially applying what he has gleaned about the causes of emotions. In other words, if he is feeling sad and would prefer to feel happy, it will help him to know some of the causes of his sadness or happiness. For example, knowing what causes his sadness can help him take steps to change the situation or his own thinking in order to reduce the sadness. Similarly, he can change the situation or his thinking in order to increase happiness. This process is, of course, emotion regulation, a topic that is discussed in detail later in the chapter.

Hiding and changing emotions serve goals that are *intra*personal, like hiding anxiety when asking someone to dance or reducing sadness by talking to a friend. In addition, masking or changing emotions also serves *inter*personal goals, such as when hiding disappointment over a gift received in order to maintain a relationship or getting psyched up so one's team does better in the game. Development of this understanding involves increases in (1) the belief that it is possible not only to change but also to control one's emotional reactions; (2) an understanding of the need for, and the advantages of, adherence to display rules; and (3) the use of both primary (problem-focused) and secondary (emotion-focused) coping strategies.

In short, children develop a relatively complex understanding of how emotions are expressed, how they occur, how they are caused, and how to change them. The complexity of emotional experience means that there is a lot to learn about emotions in the quest for emotional competence. Emotion awareness represents an important first step, but the emotion understanding factors reviewed here are critical for the later development of empathy and emotion regulation. Module 2 focuses on the learning points and activities related to these several aspects of emotion understanding.

Empathy

The capacity to respond with empathy is another key skill contributing to emotional competence (Saarni, 1999). Empathy and sympathy are two closely related words whose definitions warrant discussion. Saarni (1999) defines empathy as *feeling with* and sympathy as *feeling for*. Thus empathy is a more "involved" construct and is thought to represent a more mature form of emotional experiencing. As an example, a child is sympathetic when she feels badly for the kid in her class who is yelled at by the teacher, and she is empathic when she later talks with that kid about the experience, offering support. In other words, empathy helps one be in tune with another's situation to offer assistance.

> **empathy:** feeling with another, such that one can respond effectively to offer assistance or support.

Many scientists have noted that the development of empathy progresses through phases. First, there is *quasi-mimesis*, when a child simply responds in a "mimicking" (although not mean-spirited) manner to another's emotion. This is when, for instance, a child cries when his friend cries, not because he understands how the friend feels but because he is imitating what the friend is doing. Next, there is *emotional introjection*, when the child "walks in the other's shoes" and thus imagines himself in the other's situation. Doing so allows him to begin to know how the other is feeling. For example, if his friend is crying because her ice cream has fallen from the cone, the child might imagine himself standing there with an empty ice-cream cone. Third, there is *reverberation*. Here, the child experiences the other's feelings by remembering his own similar emotional experiences. As he watches his friend crying, he remembers times when he has lost his ice cream or had a similar "lost treat" situation. To this point, one can see that the child's experience of his friend's emotion has become more and more intense and personal. This is helpful insofar as it allows the child to know what his friend is feeling. However, the consequence of his feeling the same feeling as his friend can become problematic if his own feelings get in the way of his helping his friend. Here, the separation between sympathy and empathy is most stark. The move to real empathy, according to this definition, comes with what is called *boundaried empathy*. The child learns to create a barrier between himself and the other so that he can "feel with" without "feeling for" (and thereby risking "feeling too much"). With this sort of empathy, he is able to offer instrumental help. As the reader certainly recognizes, this boundaried empathy is the daily work of the therapist.

Many and perhaps most children experience the emotions of others with empathy to some extent, thereby promoting social relationships. Some children often have trouble recognizing the feelings of others. These children often lack the emotion awareness and understanding needed to develop empathy skills. There is a third group of children who experience personal distress in the face of the emotional experiences of others. These children often express anger or frustration when other children are emotional, sometimes reacting aggressively or punitively toward these children. Module 3 provides guidance to help children develop empathy and offers troubleshooting advice for all three problems mentioned above.

Emotion Regulation

Research on emotion regulation has increased rapidly in the last decade. As Gross and Thompson (2007) note, the scientific study of emotion regulation stems from two different theoretical approaches: the personality psychology approach, with roots in research on stress/coping, psychoanalytic study of psychological defenses, and functionalist emotion theory; and the developmental psychology approach, again with roots in functionalist theory, highlighting the development of emotion regulation via multiple factors (e.g., temperament, socialization). These two approaches have at times operated in parallel, leading to some divergence in conceptualization of the construct of emotion regulation. Fortunately, work in the past decade has focused on clarifying the construct. Although that process has not led to a definitive conceptualization, a common set of precepts has emerged.

> **emotion regulation:** "extrinsic and intrinsic processes responsible for monitoring, evaluating and modifying emotional reactions, especially their intensive and temporal features, to accomplish one's goals" (Thompson, 1994, pp. 27–28).

First, although emotion regulation is viewed as a dialectical construct, involving both emotion as a behavior regulator and emotion as a regulated phenomenon, most research emphasizes the latter. As an example, Thompson's (1994) definition is frequently referenced: "extrinsic and intrinsic processes responsible for monitoring, evaluating and modifying emotional reactions especially their intensive and temporal features, to accomplish one's goals" (pp. 27–28). Furthermore, he outlines several possible ways that emotion is regulated: (1) neurophysiological response (a brain-mediated somatic response like when, under stress, the body releases adrenaline to prepare us for fast action); (2) attentional processes (i.e., focusing attention on a particular stimulus, such as when one focuses on the finish line during a race to keep from experiencing exhaustion); (3) construals/attributions (i.e., "explaining" something that happens to oneself in a way to alter one's emotional reaction, such as attributing a team's lack of success in a game to bad luck in order to help keep spirits up); (4) access to coping resources (i.e., being able to talk or interact with a trusted person); (5) exposure to environment (i.e., when one is in a particular place that has an impact on one's emotions, like a fun party that lightens one's spirits); and (6) responses/behavior (i.e., specific behaviors one engages in to change one's feelings, such as when one chooses to engage in a reliably enjoyable activity to lift one's spirits).

A second aspect of emotion regulation is related to the distinction between control and regulation. Most theorists view emotion regulation as going beyond control, instead referring to the "dynamic ordering and adjusting" (Cole, Michel, & Teti, 1994, p. 83) of emotional behavior. Control, in contrast, is viewed as the restraint of emotional processes. Hence, most agree that emotion regulation involves more than merely stopping or reducing emotion. In fact, sometimes emotion regulation involves increasing emotional arousal (e.g., creating a positive and upbeat attitude in a car full of complaining children; cf. emotion cultivation; Fredrickson, 1998). Along these lines, emotion dysregulation is not necessarily only the lack of "control" over one's emotions, but instead regulation that is "operating in a dysfunctional manner" (Cole et al., 1994, p. 80).

A third aspect of emotion regulation involves child and environmental variables (e.g., family, culture). The transaction of child temperament and caregiver characteristics and behaviors (e.g., attachment, parenting style) in the development of emotion regulation is of particular importance (e.g., Calkins, 1994). From this perspective, emotion regulation develops largely in the context of the relationship(s) between the child and his/her parents/caregivers.

Finally, emotion regulation is viewed as an integral process in socioemotional competence and mental health. In other words, regulating one's emotions represents a critical challenge, important for both interpersonal and intrapersonal functioning.

Emotion regulation occurs in multiple ways and via a number of processes. Two different perspectives on emotion regulation are examined below: a process/functional model and a developmental model.

Process/Functional Model of Emotion Regulation

The process/functional model, introduced by Gross and Thompson (2007), identifies five categories of regulatory processes. From a behavioral perspective, these five categories involve both antecedent-focused and consequence/response-focused processes.

The first category, *situation selection*, is an antecedent-focused approach to regulation, involving the selection of situations to maximize positive emotion and minimize negative emotion. Of course, there are many ways to abuse this strategy. For example, avoiding social situations is an effective way to reduce anxiety for a shy person but is not likely to be adaptive in the long run. However, the strategy also has many benefits, especially when applied with our own long-term mental health in mind. As Gross and Thompson (2007) note, the situation selection strategy is a common one used by parents. Parents do their best to select situations that will stretch their children just enough to help them grow but not so much as to overly tax them. Situation selection, thus, also represents a strategy for which emotion socialization is critical. The strategy is used, and thereby modeled, by caregivers.

The second category, *situation modification*, is subtly different from situation selection in that it involves altering an ongoing situation rather than selecting a new situation altogether. Situation selection is an antecedent-management strategy, whereas situation modification is a response-focused strategy. For example, imagine a shy child who is going to a party. She may decide to arrive at the party early in anticipation that she will have fewer people staring at her as she enters. This would be a situation-selection (or antecedent-focused) approach. However, once she arrives at the party, imagine that the partygoers turn on the karaoke machine and start to sing. Our shy girl can try to modify the situation by offering to serve as the audience for the singers, thus reducing her distress through modifying an ongoing situation.

The third category is *attention deployment*, another response-focused strategy that involves conscious focus on certain aspects of an ongoing, emotionally charged situation. Examples of attention deployment include distraction, concentration, and even dissociation. Evidence of this strategy can be apparent in preschool-age children, although more conscious use of attention deployment strategies develops later.

The fourth category is *cognitive changes or appraisals*. A cognitive strategy is typically, although not always, a response-focused strategy. One can consider and employ multiple appraisals before, during, and after a particular situation in order to regulate emotional responses. For example, imagine a child's reaction after her swim team's loss in a meet. Cognitive appraisal can either involve downplaying the importance of the meet (e.g., "This meet was not as important as the meet we won last week against our main rival") or emphasizing good efforts (e.g., "I swam my best and actually had a personal best time"). Similar (or alternative) cognitive appraisals can be employed later (e.g., the next day at school when the swim meet results are announced and others ask about the event). These sorts of post hoc appraisals are the bread and butter of many cognitive treatment approaches for child and adolescent behavior problems; however, appraisals can also be used on the antecedent side (e.g., in advance of the next swim meet). As the meet approaches, the child can remind herself of her strong performance ("I did great at my last meet") or think positively about the potential of her teammates ("My team has practiced extra hard this week").

Obviously, these same strategies can also be used to increase negative emotion. Our swimmer could just as easily deflate her mood state by focusing on the meet's importance ("If we lose this next one we'll have no shot at the championship") or how bad her own performance was ("I lost my event and cost my team a lot of points").

The fifth and final category suggested by Gross and Thompson is *response modulation*. Response modulation occurs late in the sequence and typically involves an effort to alter the actual emotional response. An example would be a child who initially cries about something but, upon realizing that the response is not yielding the hoped-for outcome, changes tactics and goes with whining or perhaps even using words to express his feelings.

In short, the model outlined by Gross and Thompson offers numerous applications for prevention and treatment interventions, many of which are depicted in the modules that follow in this book. Although more research is needed, there is considerable evidence that children who engage in more of these emotion regulation strategies across all five categories fare better (e.g., Gross & Thompson, 2007).

Hence, teaching children to apply skills from all five categories may be a beneficial strategy.

Developmental Model of Emotion Regulation

A different, complementary view of emotion regulation focuses on the development of emotion regulation, which appears to move in Wernerian (Werner, 1957) style toward increasing sophistication and differentiation in regulation. In this brief review, I present the major milestones of emotion regulation in developmental order.

One of the earliest forms of regulation is emotion expression itself, as discussed earlier. There are several regulatory effects of expressing an emotion. First, emotion expression often has an impact on others in the environment who can offer instrumental help or support. Hence, this is a particularly important strategy early in life as we begin to get our bearings in our emotional lives. Expressing an emotion is an early step toward coming to know what that emotion is—and then what to do about it. Accordingly, emotion expression sets the stage for a number of important emotion-related processes, including emotion awareness, emotion understanding, and, of course, emotion socialization.

Another early regulation strategy involves elemental cognitive and associative learning strategies. As an example, a caretaker can soothe a crying baby just by speaking softly, even if the caretaker does nothing to "fix" the actual problem (e.g., hunger, wet diaper). The infant will have learned to associate the caregiver's voice with impending relief. Such strategies become more complex with age and language development.

Emotion expression and associative learning are probably not the first strategies most therapists and parents associate with emotion regulation. Deliberate (i.e., planful) regulation involves a goal-oriented application of emotion understanding (i.e., *doing* that stems from *knowing*); however, "doing" emotion regulation often precedes "knowing" what to do, although knowing clearly helps the doing. In fact, children will often engage in particular emotion regulation strategies of which, when asked, they claim ignorance. Hence, it is perhaps most precise to think that children learn over time to become more deliberate in their use of strategies for regulating emotions.

In the modules that make up Part II of this book, the different emotion regulation-relevant interventions described can be located in both the developmental framework and the Gross and Thompson model described here.

Emotion Socialization

The final construct to consider, emotion socialization, is critical in clinical work because many interventions for children and adolescents employ strategies that leverage emotion socialization processes. As discussed earlier in regard to emotional competence, children learn about their emotions and how to regulate them largely in social contexts. Obviously, one of the most important of these contexts, especially early in development, is the family. Most of what is known about emotion socialization is drawn from work on family emotion socialization. Before discussing parental influence on emotion socialization, it should be noted that the family obviously contributes to the child's emotion development through genetic endowment of particular temperamental styles and the resulting level of match between those styles and the caregivers' in the child's environment.

> **emotion socialization:** intentional and unintentional processes by which significant others, particularly parents, teach children about emotional knowledge and regulation.

There are several parent/family-related "nurture" effects on a child's emotion development; I discuss each briefly.

An important early contributor is the quality of the parent–child relationship and the attachment bond experienced (e.g., Calkins, 2007). A secure attachment relationship allows the parent and child to engage in open and flexible communication about a range of topics, including emotion. One of the roots for this positive transaction lies in early flexible responses to infant emotion displays, setting the stage for both a strong attachment relationship and for open communication about emotional experiences (e.g., Calkins & Fox, 2002). In other words, parents and caregivers who can avoid rigidity in their response style are more likely to promote strong emotion regulation in their children. Overall, it appears likely that a secure attachment between child and parent sets the stage for positive emotion socialization, whereas insecure attachment places a child at risk for emotion functioning difficulties.

A more direct path of emotion socialization is found in parents' efforts to manage a child's emotions. Parental soothing and/or distraction of an upset child are standard examples, but there are myriad ways that this happens. For example, a parent teaches emotional competence by engaging with her child in activities that create and maintain positive emotional states. Parents also teach this indirectly by encouraging children to participate in activities or by simply suggesting they go outside and play. In addition, parents explicitly teach children the strategy of activity selection when they explain why they are sending them outside: "You seem bored. Why don't you go out with your friend and play some ball? That might help."

As children get older and experience more cognitive sophistication, parents can engage in more elaborate emotion management strategies, including problem solving and cognitive interventions that help the child see alternative ways to think about a situation. Through these and other routes discussed next, a caregiver provides scaffolding (e.g., Denham, Mason, & Couchoud, 1995) that enables and fosters a child's emotional development.

In addition to direct management of a child's emotions, parents also socialize children through their evaluations of the child's emotional behaviors. This includes both intended emotion socialization as well as unintended emotion socialization, the latter of which occurs when parents reinforce negative emotion by attending to it, whether supportively or critically. Engaging in supportive attention can facilitate emotion regulation because such support can lead to decreases in negative emotion, thus encouraging the child to express emotion when overwhelmed; and the child also can learn that social support is an effective strategy for emotion regulation. However, supportive attending can also backfire if the child learns that attention is provided when she expresses negative emotions. Obviously, critical attention is likely to have a negative impact on a child's emotion regulation. Some interventions that focus on altering how parents communicate with children about emotions have been based around the notion of the damage done by overly critical reactions to a child's emotional reactions (e.g., Miklowitz & Goldstein, 2010; Wood & McLeod, 2007). For example, Wood and McLeod describe an approach based in part on work by Ginott (1965) and Faber and Mazlich (1995) that emphasizes the acceptance and encouragement of child emotion-related talk ("It sounds like you feel very upset about Tommy stealing your pencil"), rather than discounting or denying a child's emotional expression ("It is just a pencil. No need to get bent out of shape about it.").

Parent–child emotion conversations, as distinguished from parental reactions to child emotions, are another important way that parents socialize their children about emotions (e.g., Eisenberg, Cumberland, & Spinrad, 1998). These talks can occur during or after an emotional event, such as after a mother has just yelled angrily at her son. The mother may then talk with the son about her anger, its source, how she attempted to cope with it, and how she still loves him despite her angry feelings. Parents and children can also have more general conversations about emotions. For example, a child may hear about guilt on a TV show or read about it in a book and ask her parents what it means. The parents can then talk to their daughter about guilt and what she might do to deal with the feeling herself. These conversations can have an important normalizing effect; understanding that emotions are a normal part of being human has regulatory benefits. What's more, these emotion conversations easily lead into what Gottman has called "emotion coaching" sessions, wherein the parent offers strategies for the child to try in future emotional situations (e.g., Gottman, Katz, & Hooven, 1996). Coaching sessions provide both the opportunity for children to see parents model how to handle feeling and for children to rehearse handling emotions differently in a "practice" situation.

Furthermore, the overall emotional climate of the family has an effect on a child's emotion development. Families vary widely in terms of which emotions are acceptable to express, who can express them, and how they can be expressed. Frequent and intense expression of negative emotion by family members is linked to poor outcomes. Parental emotion expression and parental regulation of their own emotions represent key learning opportunities, with parents serving as models for methods of experiencing and dealing with feelings. To the extent that parents are aware of and make use of these opportunities, it bodes well for the emotion socialization of the child.

In summary, there are several pathways through which emotion socialization occurs in the family, including parent–child attachment, direct parent teaching of emotion regulation, and parent–child emotion conversations. Similar processes take place in extrafamilial emotion socialization, although these other influences (e.g., peer, teacher) are rarely studied. Because parents and caregivers can be involved in any of the modules described later in the book, it is fair to say that all of the modules are influenced by the important concept of emotion socialization.

OTHER KEY CONCEPTS: INDIVIDUAL DIFFERENCES AND TEMPERAMENT

Two final topics warrant brief discussion here: individual differences in emotional development and temperament.

Individual Differences

Although individual differences and diversity are discussed in more detail in Chapter 6, it is worth noting here that gender and culture influence emotional development in ways therapists should be aware of and look out for.

Gender

Evidence suggests that boys believe emotion should be expressed less than girls do, implying a perceived need on the part of boys more than girls to regulate their emotional expression (e.g., Underwood, 1997). However, things become a bit murkier when boys and girls are asked about the consequences of emotional expression. Some studies show that girls expect more negative reactions from peers than boys for expressing emotion, whereas other studies have found that boys have the more negative expectation (e.g., Underwood, 1997; Zeman & Shipman, 1997). In short, although gender may influence children's perceptions about the need to regulate and the consequences of regulating their emotions, the gender effect appears to be a nuanced one, possibly depending on contextual factors.

Research on gender differences in empathy suggests that there is some nuance here too. For example, much research has suggested that females are more empathic than males (e.g., Eisenberg & Lennon, 1983; Rueckert & Naybar, 2008). However, the finding is more robust when the method for assessing empathy is self-report (e.g., Eisenberg & Lennon, 1983). That is, when asked, girls say that they experience more empathy than boys do. However, systematic observations of children reveal no such gender difference on actual empathy behavior (e.g., Eisenberg &

Lennon, 1983). Thus it's possibile that boys and girls may be similarly empathic and the real difference is that girls are more likely to talk about it.

Culture

The reader will no doubt intuit that not all cultures share the same views on emotion expression and regulation. Unfortunately, there are relatively few studies examining individual differences in emotional development related to culture. Ultimately, though, more empirical work is needed to study how culture affects emotional development. A set of programmatic studies conducted by Weisz and colleagues (Weisz, Suwanlert, Chaiyasit, Weiss, et al., 1987; Weisz et al., 1988) on culture and psychopathology has implications for understanding cultural differences on emotion processes. The research examined differences between children in the United States and children in Thailand across a number of dimensions from the perspectives of the children, their parents, and their teachers. One study found cultural differences between the two groups when children and their parents were asked about the children's coping methods and coping goal differences (i.e., their emotion regulation). Specifically, Thai children engaged in more covert coping in situations involving adult authority figures, making them less likely to overtly express their emotions in front of adults in authority. In addition, Thai children reported they were more likely than U.S. children to try to change how they thought about a situation (vs. trying to change the situation) when faced with separation from a caregiver. U.S. children, on the other hand, were more likely to try to change how they thought about the situation (vs. trying to change the situation) when they experienced a physical injury.

There are a few points to make here. One cultural difference between the United States and Thailand is that the U.S. culture is considered *individualistic,* whereas Thai culture is considered *collectivistic.* In an individualistic culture, children's emotional expression may be viewed as a means for expressing individuality and thus may be supported and even encouraged. However, in a collectivist culture oriented toward the common good, restraining emotional expression may be highly valued. A second point is that certain cultures "permit" emotional expression in some situations and not in others. For example, some Asian cultures are more supportive of expressing physical versus emotional pain, a fact that may result in Asian Americans being more willing to complain of physical problems than mental health problems (e.g., Matsumoto, 2001).

Temperament

The processes described in this chapter, which lead to the development of emotional competence, occur in individuals who are all born with different emotional predilections. The number of supposed temperamental characteristics varies across studies and also is thought to vary across development. However, a few temperamental characteristics are discussed here because of their particular relevance to emotion.

First, there is *behavioral inhibition*, or the tendency to react to novel stimuli with extreme inhibition. Jerome Kagan, Joseph Biederman, and their colleagues at Massachusetts General Hospital and Harvard University have provided strong evidence that inhibited temperament is stable and the style is associated with later internalizing disorders (e.g., anxiety disorders; Biederman, et al., 1993; Kagan, Snidman, Arcus, & Reznick, 1994). They have also suggested that other temperament patterns (e.g., uninhibited) may be associated with externalizing disorders (e.g., Schwartz, Snidman, & Kagan, 1996).

Along similar lines, Derryberry and Reed (1994) posited two temperamental patterns that may be vulnerabilities for the development of psychopathology. First, they described a *reward/approach* orientation that may create a vulnerability to impulsivity-related disorders. Second, they described a *punishment/avoidance orientation* that may place a child at risk for developing an anxiety disorder.

A final temperamental characteristic, *emotional intensity*, is the tendency to have extreme emotional reactions (or not). Eisenberg and colleagues have studied the relations among emotional intensity, emotion regulation, and social adjustment, noting that elevated levels of negative emotional intensity (i.e., negative emotions like anger, sadness, or fear) represent a risk factor, while high general and positive emotional intensities are also linked to negative outcomes (e.g., Eisenberg et al., 1996). Based on their findings, Eisenberg and colleagues have posited that moderate emotional intensity relates to positive outcome (e.g., social adjustment; e.g., Eisenberg et al., 1997).

CONCLUSION

The study of emotion has emerged as a significant field in the 21st century. In this chapter, several important emotion-related constructs were defined and discussed as a prelude to the focus on the treatment strategies described in Part II of the book. Overall, the modules are guided by the model of emotional competence described by Saarni, emphasizing the development of several related but distinct skills that foster optimal functioning and adaptation.

CHAPTER 3

Emotion-Related Assessment

This chapter serves two purposes. First, it refreshes the reader's memory on some core assessment principles. Second, it describes methods used to assess emotion-related competencies.

Almost all of the evidence base for psychological treatments comes from studies that applied strong assessment before treatment. These studies rely on extensive assessments using measures that possess what is called "strong psychometrics," meaning that the instruments have been studied extensively and have been found to perform reliably and provide a valid assessment. Thus, because the focus of this book is psychological treatment interventions, rigorous assessment is strongly recommended before using any of strategies described in the book.

THE PURPOSES OF ASSESSMENT

Assessment is an activity performed to inform a plan. In mental health, the plan may include a psychological treatment plan, educational placement, out-of-home placement (e.g., foster home, residential treatment center), or the use of medication. The plan is based on the hypothesis of the person implementing the plan, which is itself based on her assessment of the situation—that is, her hypotheses about why problems exist and persist for the client. Sometimes, very little assessment is needed. For example, a family may present to treatment with a clearly articulated understanding of the problem and its causes. In such cases, the therapist may be able to proceed with very little additional assessment beyond the family's own observations. However, if a plan based on these observations fails, the therapist might conclude that the information available to the family was insufficient: their hypotheses about how to resolve things were incorrect or incomplete. If treatment fails in a case like this, formal assessment might be warranted.

Of course, it is rare in clinical practice to have a family present to treatment with a comprehensive and largely accurate understanding of the problems facing their child. Instead, families usually have many questions and much uncertainty. Often, the main reason for families to seek out a therapist is to get an answer to the question "What is wrong with my child?"

Assessment can be used to answer four separate but related questions, each of which are discussed below:

1. Is more assessment needed?
2. Is any intervention warranted?
3. What are the client's specific problems, and which treatments will best address those problems?
4. How well is the intervention is working?

Is More Assessment Needed?

This question is not always part of a typical clinical assessment because a referral may imply that the family already knows they want more assessment. But there are times when a therapist may be asked to screen a particular child or perhaps even a classroom full of them. As such, screening assessments answer the question "Is more assessment needed?" Screenings are typically brief and administered to large groups of potential clients/patients. Although a screening will not provide enough information to determine the presence of a diagnosis or detail the scope of a problem, such measures may be incorporated into more thorough, comprehensive assessments that take place later. Screening measures can be administered individually to identify possible foci for comprehensive assessments or to large groups to identify need for services or further assessment (e.g., administering a measure of depression to students at a local school).

Is Any Intervention Warranted?

This question can arise either after a positive screening result or when a family refers a child to a clinic or provider, asking for an opinion about whether the child needs behavioral health services. When someone comes through the door of a mental health clinic, both parties may assume that mental health treatment will be recommended. However, as anyone with a cold who has gone to a primary care doctor can attest, there are times when good assessment leads a professional to conclude: "What is ailing you can be 'cured' without formal treatment." Such instances in mental health are certainly rare, though, and the most common situation is that a family has waited a long (and agonizing) time before concluding that some intervention may be needed. Still, it is worth underscoring that one of the purposes of assessment is to determine whether a child's problems warrant intervention.

To make this determination, the therapist should identify whether the problems are developmentally inappropriate in the observed context, and whether the problems cause sufficient distress or interference to merit formally addressing them in some way. The first part of this decision is often guided by measures of the problem areas identified by the family. The therapist should ask herself, "Is the intensity or severity of the problem out of the range of what is developmentally normative?" Using measures with strong psychometrics (e.g., reliability, validity, norms) supports the endeavor by increasing confidence in the conclusions reached. The topic of measures, psychometrics, and norms will be revisited shortly.

The second part of this decision is informed by a measure related not to a specific problem area (or areas) per se, but to the functional consequences of those problems. For example, failure to attend school, lack of friends, feelings of extreme distress, and academic impairment are all indicators of possible need for treatment and are not always assessed solely by measures that gauge symptoms. Thus the therapist must also consider using measures that tap functional consequences of problem areas.

What Are the Client's Specific Problems, and Which Treatments Will Best Address Those Problems?

The third question answered is only asked if the answer to the second question was yes, and intervention is, in fact, warranted. The measures used to inform problem identification and treatment selection will vary. For instance, the therapist could collect diagnostic and symptomatic information by interviewing the family; conduct structured or semistructured observations of the family in a variety of contexts (e.g., office, school, home); or gather information from significant others in the family's life (e.g., teachers, coaches). Further discussion of these methods follows shortly, but suffice it to say here that this third question—what the focus of treatment shall be—may involve the most comprehensive and time-consuming effort from the provider. In our clinic at VCU, we generally rely not only on a set of measures and interviews but also on the functional assessment process described in Chapter 4. Furthermore, as underscored in that chapter and in Chapter 5, the question of *focus* is not answered definitively at the outset. As information changes during treatment, the focus may shift, become clearer, or sometimes become murkier. Thus the process of deciding how and where to focus treatment is ongoing.

How Well Is the Intervention Working?

The fourth question is as important as the first three, although it is the one most often neglected. Assessment is also used to gauge the ongoing effects of a plan or intervention. The therapist should collect data to answer questions like "Is the plan working? Is the child's functioning improving?" The measurement strategies needed for this purpose are ideally brief and focused, to maximize the likelihood of frequent feedback. For example, a family whose son has regular emotional outbursts may report the number of these outbursts weekly or, to focus on the positive opposite, they may report on the number of times the child was able to regulate his emotional response in a challenging situation. In addition to teaching the family to gather such information weekly, the therapist can also use a standardized measure of behavior on a less frequent basis to see whether treatment gains are generalizing beyond an area of particular focus, as well as to ensure that the client's problems have not simply "moved" to another domain.

With the general purposes of assessment reviewed, the last section of the chapter discusses several tools related to the assessment of emotion-related constructs.

EMOTION ASSESSMENT

Measurement specific to emotion is less common than measurement of clinical phenomena, particularly clinical symptoms. As discussed in Chapter 2, emotion has only recently become a common target of scientific study, and so development of measurement tools for emotion lags behind measurement in other areas. An additional difficulty in taking emotion measurements with children specifically is that developmental issues can interfere with clients' abilities to respond to certain questions about their feelings. While measuring children's emotional competencies by asking them directly is perhaps the best choice, therapists must keep in mind that a child's take on her emotional competence may be wrong or incomplete. Multimethod measurement—using more than one measure for the same concept and, ideally, more than one reporter—should help offset this problem.

Before reviewing specific emotion measures, a few prefatory issues warrant comment. First, measurement of emotion must consider the developmental status of the child in question. There is some scientific evidence to suggest that asking children under the age of 6 about their emotions may be an exercise in futility (Lewis, Haviland-Jones, & Barrett, 2008). Of course, there are some extraordinary 5-year-olds who can talk about their emotions just as there are some 14-year-olds who do not seem able to do so. An age-based rule of thumb should be applied flexibly.

In addition, self-report measures often rely on rating scales. For example, a child may be asked to rate his frequency of use of a specific emotion regulation strategy on a scale from 1 to 7, with each number having a descriptor associated with it. Again, there are developmental differences associated with children being able to make this sort of judgment.

Finally, children are particularly susceptible to the social desirability bias. In other words, children may respond to interviews or questionnaires according to their perception of what is correct or socially desirable rather than replying with true answers. Adults are prone to this response style as well, but unlike adults in most clinical assessment situations, children have rarely asked to be assessed. As such, their motivation to respond honestly and completely is perhaps best described as mixed.

The following section describes measures for two of the most often studied emotion related constructs: *emotion understanding* and *emotion regulation*. Although the focus is primarily on self-report measures, other methods are described as well, reflecting the importance of multimethod measurement.

Emotion Understanding Measures

Measurements of emotion understanding are designed to gauge how well children grasp specific emotion-related concepts (e.g., knowing that there are many different kinds of feelings, that each has a particular set of associated physiological responses, and that each can be triggered by a variety of internal and external events). Typically, measurement of emotion understanding is done in an interview format because it removes the need for literacy, permits an interviewer to adjust questions to a child's developmental level, and allows for follow-up and clarifying questions; however, questionnaires have also been used to measure emotion understanding. Two interviews and one questionnaire with good psychometric evidence supporting them are described here.

Interviews

The Emotional Understanding Interview (EUI; Cassidy, Parke, Butkovsky, & Braungart, 1992) involves showing the child a picture of a same-sex peer who is expressing one of four emotions (i.e., anger, sadness, happiness, and fear). The child is then asked a series of open-ended questions about the picture, with questions falling into five categories tapping different aspects of emotion understanding: (1) identification of emotion (e.g., "How do you think this child is feeling?"); (2) experience of emotion (e.g., "Do you ever feel like this?"); (3) causes of emotion (e.g., "What kinds of things make you feel this way?"); (4) expression of emotion, (e.g., "When you feel this way, do you let other people know how you feel?"); and (5) action responses to emotional displays (e.g., "If you saw another kid looking this way, what would you do?"). Each response is scored as either "yes" or "no." "Yes" means the child appears to understand that particular aspect of emotion, and "no" means the child does not appear to understand. The therapist might opt to include pictures for all four emotions, or shorten the assessment by selecting only certain pictures. Scores are summed to produce a total score, as well as a score for each of the four emotions.

The Kusche Affective Interview—Revised (KAI-R; Kusché, Bielke, & Greenberg, 1988) is a longer and more comprehensive tool used to gauge emotion understanding. The KAI-R consists of a series of open-ended questions, divided into several sections. The first section assesses knowledge of emotion words; the child is asked to list as many emotions as she knows. The second section tests knowledge about possible cues for emotions (e.g., situational cues, facial cues, internal cues). Specifically, children are asked, "How do you know when you are feeling . . . ?" for 10 emotions (e.g., happy, sad, mad, scared, love, proud, guilty, jealous, nervous, lonely); they are prompted to respond to each question with as many cues as they can think of. The third section assesses understanding of multiple emotion combinations—that is, children are asked whether one can feel more than one feeling at the same time, and specific combinations are queried (e.g., sad and mad; happy and sad; calm and nervous; love and anger). The fourth section assesses knowledge of the idea that feelings can be hidden (e.g., "How do you hide your feelings from others? How do others hide their feelings from you?"). The fifth section assesses knowledge about the idea that emotions can change (e.g., "Can you change your feelings? How?"). Other sections assess beliefs about emotions, including, for example, whether animals experience emotions.

Scoring for the KAI-R is more complex than for the EUI; responses are coded using a system that estimates the relative developmental level of each response. For example, some responses are scored using a 0 to 3 scale, with 0 reflecting a very low level of understanding and 3 representing the highest level of understanding. Scores are assigned across the different sections so that a child might score highly (e.g., 3) on emotion cues knowledge, for example, but lower on knowledge about changing emotions.

Questionnaire

The Emotion Expression Scale for Children (EESC; Penza-Clyve & Zeman, 2002) is a 16-item questionnaire. Children respond using a 5-point scale on which 1 means not at all true, 3 means somewhat true, and 5 means extremely true. There are actually two separate scales in the measure: poor awareness and expressive reluctance. The poor awareness scale has items like "I often do not know how I am feeling" and "I have feelings that I can't figure out." The expressive reluctance scale has items like "I prefer to keep my feelings to myself" and "When I get upset, I am afraid to show it." Although the measure is designed as a questionnaire, it could also be given as an interview. Furthermore, there is a version of the measure that parents can complete about their children. The measure has the advantage of being brief and easily and privately completed; however, it does not capture a child's emotion understanding as broadly as either of the interviews described above. In addition, the expressive reluctance scale is perhaps not really a gauge of emotion understanding so much as a gauge of emotion expression (or lack thereof).

Although other measures exist for emotion understanding, the three described here have the most evidence supporting their use. All were developed with research purposes in mind. The interviews in particular lend themselves nicely to clinical work with children. Therapists can even use them without the formal scoring procedures as a way to begin talking to a child about feelings. All three measures are available from the authors (their e-mail addresses are at the end of this chapter).

Emotion Regulation Measures

Measurement of emotion regulation has received more attention than measurement of emotion understanding, and as a result, there are more emotion regulation measures available. For the purposes of the book, measures that gauge coping more broadly were not included, although there is important overlap with coping and emotion regulation, as discussed in Chapter 2. Emotion regulation measures have tended to be either questionnaires or observational procedures. Two questionnaires and two observational paradigms are described below.

Questionnaires

Janice Zeman and her colleagues at the University of Maine and, more recently, at The College of William and Mary, have developed a set of emotion regulation measures called the Children's Emotion Management Scales (CEMS; e.g., Zeman, Shipman, & Suveg, 2002). Currently, there are separate measures for three emotions—anger, sadness, and worry—and each measure has the same three factors: (1) *inhibition*, associated with suppression of emotional expression (e.g., "I hide my sadness/anger/worry"); (2) *dysregulated expression*, the outward expression of emotion in a dysregulated manner (e.g., "I lose my temper when I am angry"; "I whine/fuss about what is making me sad"); and (3) *coping*, associated with strategies such as behavioral distraction and social support (e.g., "I talk to someone until I feel better").

Another questionnaire is the Emotion Regulation Checklist (Shields & Cicchetti, 1997). This 24-item questionnaire is completed by parents and uses a 4-point scale to assess caregivers' perceptions of their children's abilities to regulate emotion. The questionnaire contains two scales: (1) *emotion regulation*, which assesses the situational appropriateness of affective displays, empathy, and emotional self-awareness (e.g., "Is empathic toward others"); and (2) *lability/negativity*, which assesses mood lability, lack of flexibility, dysregulated negative affect, and inappropriate affective displays (e.g., "Is prone to angry outbursts").

Observational Measures

From a commonsense vantage, measuring emotion regulation should involve more than just how well a child can "talk the talk." And of course, researchers have developed tools to see whether they can "walk the walk" as well. The observational measures developed have tended to be structured ones. One example is the *disappointing gift paradigm* (Cole, 1986; Saarni, 1984). In this situation, the child completes some tasks with a researcher. Before embarking on the tasks, the child is promised a prize in exchange for his cooperation. Afterward, the child is presented with a broken toy as the prize, and his emotional reaction is recorded and later coded to gauge how well he can regulate disappointment. The paradigm is built on the finding that even young children have learned that they need to hide their disappointment in some situations.

A second observational paradigm used to gauge emotion regulation has been called the *anger simulation* paradigm (Cummings, Hennessy, Rabideau, & Cicchetti, 1994). In one variant, a child and her caregiver are completing forms in the same room but at different tables. After a period of time, the researcher approaches the caregiver to check in and see how things are going. The researcher becomes angry that the caregiver has not made "adequate progress" and talks in an angry tone with the caregiver about how the researcher's time is valuable. During this experience, the child is being observed either through a one-way mirror or else via video recording. Here, the goal is to observe how the child copes with the anger being expressed toward her caregiver.

A few notes about the anger simulation paradigm. First, this paradigm is an example of deception research insofar as the researcher's anger is contrived. In this case, the caregiver is in on the deception as well, and the child is informed of the deception as soon as the observation is complete and is given time to discuss any feelings that she experienced. Deception studies are controversial, even when handled responsibly. No one likes to be tricked. Most therapists will not find this approach useful or appropriate without considerable thought and planning.

Observing emotion regulation can provide information that would be hard to obtain otherwise, and clinicians should consider how to create opportunities for such observation in their work with clients. Most clinicians will note that they are often privy to a number of situations in which emotion regulation can be gauged during regular therapy sessions. Indeed, impromptu emotion regulation situations are common in clinical practice. Although appealing for the ease with which they can be implemented, impromptu emotion regulation situations have threats to internal validity. In plain terms, there are often many different variables that influence behavior. When measuring the effect of a situation on another variable (like emotion regulation), the aim is to standardize as many as possible of the other variables (called *nuisance variables*) that can influence the target variable. This allows the researcher to feel confident that what is observed is primarily the result of the situation that has been contrived. When observing impromptu situations, the therapist often does not have control over, or even knowledge of, other variables that might influence the client's reactions.

Thus there are advantages to following a standard protocol like one of the questionnaires or observational measures described earlier. If a clinician applies the principle of standardization to her assessment, she will build up a database of responses that will make it easier to differentiate unusual responses from usual responses.

CONCLUSION

Entire textbooks are written on the topic of assessment (e.g., Mash & Barkley, 2007), and much more comprehensive chapters have been written on the topic of emotion-related assessments. Perhaps the most notable emotion-related assessments omitted from this chapter are brain imaging tools. As described in Chapter 2, the science of emotion is growing rapidly, largely propelled by neuroscience research. However, the impracticality of using an MRI in regular clinical practice warrants a focus on more traditional measures. The emotion-related assessments described here can be used (1) as part of an assessment process to help guide the sort of treatment planning described in the next two chapters, (2) to determine the potential applicability of the treatment modules that comprise the second part of this book, and (3) as important indicators of treatment progress.

To contact the emotion measure developers about acquiring their measures, use the contact information below.

Emotion Understanding Interview: Dr. Jude Cassidy: *jcassidy@psyc.umd.edu*

Kusche Affective Interview—Revised: Dr. Mark Greenberg: *mxg47@psu.edu*

Emotion Expression Scale for Children: Dr. Janice Zeman: *jzeman@wm.edu*

Emotion Management Scales: Dr. Janice Zeman: *jzeman@wm.edu*

Emotion Regulation Checklist: Dr. Dante Cicchetti: *cicchett@umn.edu*

CHAPTER 4

Case Conceptualization

Using Functional Analysis to Define Problems and Identify Targets for Intervention

Readers might question why a book on emotion interventions requires an entire chapter on functional analysis. The answer is that without good assessment practices, there can be no guarantee of quality treatment. Broadly speaking, this chapter will (1) define functional assessment and give background information supporting its importance to good assessment practice, (2) teach readers how to incorporate it into their practice, and (3) demonstrate its power and utility in clinical work, both in general and when using emotion-informed interventions. More specifically, this chapter will delineate a functional assessment model and describe how functional assessment can help with treatment planning, using two extended case examples as illustrations. Although functional assessment will be covered in some depth, interested readers are referred to other resources listed at the end of the chapter for a more thorough discussion.

DIAGNOSIS-DRIVEN VERSUS FUNCTIONAL-ANALYSIS-DRIVEN ASSESSMENT

As the mental health field has moved toward evidence-based treatments, programs, and practices, there has been an increasing reliance on the child's diagnosis (using the *Diagnostic and Statistical Manual of Mental Disorders* [DSM]) as the primary tool for assessment and treatment planning. Indeed, many evidence-based treatments (EBTs) are designed and tested for children meeting specific DSM diagnostic categories. The focus on the DSM has had great benefits for treatment, with the focus on discrete DSM categories for treatment development and testing leading to better treatment outcomes for many children and adolescents. However, many scientists and clinicians have lamented the limitations inherent to a DSM focus. Prominent among those limitations is the fact that many children who present for treatment meet the criteria for not just one but for several DSM disorders. If that's the case, how should a therapist proceed? Does sequential treatment using multiple treatment programs make sense, for example? Is it possible to conduct multiple treatment programs concurrently? Can and should treatment programs be designed for all of the various possible combinations of diagnoses? There are no clear answers to these questions.

Another limitation of the DSM-focused approach is that some children do not meet the criteria for any DSM disorders, and yet they present for treatment (Jensen & Weisz, 2002). How does a mental health system address these children—triage them out? If not, how should a therapist select treatment, given that there are not treatment programs for "no diagnosis"? These two examples, on different ends of the diagnostic continuum, demonstrate that reliance on the DSM alone is certain to create problems in planning treatment for children and adolescents. One possible remedy for these problems is the use of behavioral assessment and functional analysis.

Broadly speaking, functional analysis[1] (FA) is a process used to posit a set of hypotheses about why a particular behavior or set of behaviors is occurring and being maintained. It is important to note that functional analysis or any other behavioral assessment is not necessarily a replacement for a DSM-based assessment. A therapist need not choose between them; they are not mutually exclusive. In fact, using the two approaches together has some distinct advantages.

One of the largest benefits of using FA is that it permits a high degree of individualization of treatment. In this way, using FA is a remedy for those worried that some treatment approaches force clients into cookie-cutter conceptualizations. Indeed, using FA requires the therapist to create a *de novo* conceptualization for each case. Furthermore, FA requires that the therapist regularly revisit the conceptualization. As a result, the therapist's thinking about the client remains fresh and responsive to changes and developments. FA derives from a behavioral (and cognitive-behavioral) theoretical background. However, it is possible to apply the approach from other theoretical orientations.

---

[1] My understanding of functional analysis draws heavily from work by Henggeler, Schoenwald, Borduin, Rowland, & Cunningham (2009), Persons (2008), and Freeman and Miller (2002).

CONCEPTUAL BACKGROUND

Before proceeding to the description of the FA process, some readers may be interested in a quick lesson (or refresher) on the main theories from which FA has been drawn. Taken together, the three learning pathways described below (classical conditioning, operant conditioning, and social learning theory) represent fruitful places to look for hypotheses in conceptualizing a case using functional analysis.

Classical conditioning refers to the fact that learning sometimes occurs through the pairing of some (often innocuous) new stimulus with another stimulus that produces what is called an unconditioned response. Through pairing, a person comes to associate the new stimulus with the unconditioned one, such that simply presenting the new stimulus produces the response heretofore produced by the unconditioned stimulus. Examples abound in clinical work, such as a child who does not like going to a particular location (a room in the house or a certain street in the neighborhood) because it was inadvertently paired with a traumatic experience like physical or sexual abuse.

Operant conditioning represents a form of learning focused on the consequence of a behavior, be it a reward or punishment. Rewards or reinforcement improve the probability that the behavior preceding the reward will increase in frequency, whereas punishments have the opposite effect. For example, when a child follows a parental direction, praise (and other forms of reinforcement) will make it more likely that he repeats the compliant behavior. Many behavioral and cognitive-behavioral interventions are based, in part, on principles from operant conditioning theory.

Finally, *social learning theory* posits that learning occurs not only through direct experiences but also through observation of others' experiences. Particularly noteworthy are those observed experiences that yield rewards or punishments. Observing another child receiving attention from a teacher or parent because she is whining may suggest the whining strategy is worthwhile to try when seeking attention.

With the background out of the way, the functional analytic model will now be described in detail.

THE FUNCTIONAL ANALYTIC MODEL

Functional analysis, as noted earlier, is a process used to posit a set of hypotheses about why a particular behavior or set of behaviors is occurring and being maintained. There are four steps, and each is discussed in turn:

1. Problem identification.
2. Proximal driver nomination (i.e., identification of contributing factors to the problem behavior that occur "near" in time to the problem behavior).

3. Contextual/situational information gathering (i.e., identification of settings or people that make the problem behavior more likely).
4. Distal driver nomination (i.e., identification of factors that occurred in the past but that still appear to contribute to the problem behavior).

Step 1. Problem Identification

This first step is perhaps the most important, and it can be the most difficult. The challenge is not in identifying problems, as those typically abound in one's caseload. Instead, the difficulty comes in choosing which problems are most pressing, given that there are often so many problems for some cases. The goal of Step 1 is to generate a *brief and simple* list of *specific and behaviorally operationalized, potentially changeable* problems. A look at each of those italicized words more closely is warranted.

Brief and simple should remind the therapist to avoid creating a list of problems that reads like the grocery list of a large family with an empty refrigerator. Most clinical work requires a focus on a small set of issues, even in the context of a host of problems. It is hard to fix everything at once. Therapists should look for relations and overlaps among the problems, thereby increasing the potential scope of the treatment's impact while simultaneously reining in its focus to a more manageable number of potential foci. Finally, considering the goals of the client and family as compared to the therapist's own judgments and perceptions can often winnow down the number of problems. It may be true that one family's communication style is not the most pleasing, and by working toward changes in the style one might indeed improve the family's quality of life. However, it may also be true that the family has little or no interest in making changes in that domain. In such a case, the "family communication" problem may be on a separate therapist wish list—items that can be attended to once the more pressing (and perhaps more pertinent) problems are addressed. In general, aiming for three to five problems is a good rule of thumb. By keeping the number as small as possible, the odds of successfully addressing those problems is increased, thereby reinforcing the client (who is glad to have made progress) and the therapist (who experiences a welcome sense of success).

Specific and behaviorally operationalized is a mouthful and is also often the most difficult aspect of undertaking FA despite the relatively simple idea that the more clearly defined in behavioral terms the problem is, the better FA will work. Specific, behaviorally operationalized problems possess a few common characteristics.

First, they are specific and not global, meaning they reference particular behaviors or patterns of behavior, like fighting with peers in school or arguing with one's mother about the house rules. Broad problems, by contrast, might include aggression or oppositional behavior.

Second, the problems should be observable—that is, the problems should be behaviors that can be witnessed by others or reliably inferred and/or reported on by the client. Thus a problem like "client has poor self-esteem" is not as strong as "client rarely engages in new activities" or "client regularly expresses lack of self-confidence" because self-esteem is not directly observable.

Third, the problems should be *potentially changeable*. That may sound odd at first; after all, therapists are in the change business, so identifying behaviors that can change should be easy. However, sometimes clients are grappling with problems that have little chance of changing much. One example of a problem that might not be changeable is "client has attention-deficit/hyperactivity disorder (ADHD)." Clearly, ADHD poses numerous challenges to children and their families, and it might be tempting to add that to the list.

Let's take a closer look using the criteria just discussed for the problem "client has ADHD."

Is It Brief and Simple?

ADHD is brief (i.e., not wordy) but *not* simple, as it refers to a DSM diagnosis composed of more than a dozen symptoms across two broad categories of symptoms: inattention and hyperactivity/impulsivity. To meet DSM criteria, a child needs only six of those symptoms. Thus it is possible that two children with ADHD could have zero symptom overlap and thus would appear quite different from each other despite both meeting criteria for the same disorder. Hence, using ADHD in the problem area is not simple enough.

Is It Specific and Observable?

ADHD is not, strictly speaking, observable, although many people believe they know it when they see it; however, not everyone agrees on what ADHD *looks like*. As noted already, ADHD comprises many symptoms and thus varies in its presentation within and between children. Furthermore, some of the symptoms of ADHD contain imprecise language that makes it possible for different observers to report different things (e.g., the criterion "often easily distractible" may be viewed differently by teachers and parents). Finally, some of the symptoms of ADHD overlap with other problems and diagnoses, further complicating the issue of reliable measurement. How does one know, for example, whether the parent is reporting on distractibility due to ADHD rather than distractibility due to anxiety or fatigue?

Is It Potentially Changeable?

One could use remission of diagnosis as an indicator. Using DSM, though, a child who is diagnosis-free may still experience five problematic symptoms. Furthermore, it is worth asking: Is remission really a reasonable goal? Is it really the parent's goal?

Solution

Better, more realistic targets for a client with ADHD might include the reduction or elimination of impulsive acts in the classroom (or at home or with the client's sister), fewer tantrums at home (or school), or increased compliance with verbal requests from parents or teachers.

Step 2. Proximal Driver Nomination

Once the list of problems has been defined, the therapist is ready to identify proximal drivers. The discussion here uses the terminology consistent with Henggeler et al. (2009) in their book on multisystemic therapy. Drivers are the factors that "drive" or determine (in part) the problematic behaviors. Proximal drivers are potential factors influencing the problem behavior occurring very near in time to the problem behavior. It is worth noting that FA necessarily involves somewhat arbitrary labeling. A different analysis could certainly lead to a different organization, in which one person's problem is another person's driver. For example, assessment may suggest that the client's problem is avoiding conversation with peers at school, and that a relevant driver is negative self-talk (i.e., the client saying bad things about her ability to talk with her peers). An alternative conceptualization could posit that negative self-talk is the problem and then seek to identify drivers for it. FA is not about creating a definitive scientific theory about the nature of problematic behavior. Rather, FA is the application of scientific thinking that helps therapists understand how a given problem might be caused and maintained. It represents a guess and is best viewed (and used) as a means to an end—treatment planning—rather than a definitive theoretical statement about the etiology of a psychiatric disorder.

Proximal driver identification is facilitated by remembering the behavioral ABCs, in which A = antecedents, B = behavior, and C = consequences. Many drivers for problematic behaviors can be found in the world of the antecedents. That is why the question "What was happening right before the [insert problem here] happened?" is such a good one. Some antecedents may be conditioned stimuli; for example, being in the room where abuse took place can trigger flashbacks or aggressive outbursts. Other antecedents can serve as triggers for behaviors learned via operant conditioning; for example, when the mother's increasingly loud yelling leads to an escalation in the child's problem behavior. An examination of the history may reveal that the loudest yeller in the family gets his or her way. In this example, one could also replace "mother's increasingly loud yelling" with "mother's verbal ambivalence" and tell a similar story.

Other potentially important antecedents are harder to observe directly and require someone to articulate them. Imagine a girl who, before engaging in cutting behaviors, engages in negative self-talk. Imagine that she says to herself, "I am such a loser—everybody hates me." The event is not observable, making self-deprecating self-talk a poor choice for proximal driver nomination unless the therapist can get the client to verbalize her thoughts, thereby making them somewhat observable. If true, of course, the self-talk may be highly relevant to the problematic behavior, but a mere guess on the therapist's part is not enough to warrant its inclusion as a proximal driver.

Next on the tour of the ABCs would normally be the B. However, the B in the functional analytic process is the problematic behavior discussed earlier and does not warrant additional discussion here. Thus it is time to discuss the C, or consequences. Identifying consequences can sometimes be an easier task than identifying problems; people tend to have a better memory for what happened after a problem because the prominence of the problem leads them to start paying more attention. Thinking rather simply about consequences, consider the responses to a certain behavior that either rewarded or punished it. Take the classic example of the child in the supermarket begging for a candy bar. If the begging is viewed as the behavior, a lot rides on what the parent does for the consequence. If the parent gives in after a long begging session and provides the candy bar, the child is rewarded for begging (and the parent is rewarded for giving the candy bar because the child stops begging).

Similarly, one can consider the absence of reward from the consequence point of view. Imagine a child who has engaged in a positive behavior, like clearing the table after dinner without being asked. Sometimes (often?), parents will forget to reward a child for doing something like this. Now consider the parents' omission of a reward for the positive behavior in light of how often they pay attention to "bad" behaviors like whining or forgetting to clear the table, and the importance of the reward (and its absence) becomes clearer. To contemplate all relevant consequences, one needs to think of rewards (or punishments) given as well as those *not* given.

Another common consequence to consider is negative reinforcement, which occurs when an unpleasant stimulus is removed after a behavior has occurred. For example, when a person hits the snooze button in the morning, that action is negatively reinforced because the buzzer or radio noise ceases (that is, assuming the person does not like her sleep interrupted by a loud sound). A prisoner who receives a few years off his sentence for good behavior is also being negatively reinforced. A child may be negatively reinforced for throwing a tantrum because the tantrum leads to her not having to complete a chore or do her homework.

As with the antecedent side, the therapist can also posit internal (e.g., cognitive) consequences, although as before, these ought to be used tentatively given the difficulty inherent in observing them. However, it is certainly possible that what a client says to himself after he does something could have an impact on whether he repeats that behavior. For example, if a child focuses on how he always messes up when trying something new (e.g., playing basketball), and if afterward he recounts to himself all of his many mistakes, he may be less inclined to try that behavior in the future. Although a therapist may cautiously posit internal consequences, confidence in their applicability increases notably when what the client or other person reports corroborates the therapist's hypothesis.

In short, identifying proximal drivers involves thinking through the ABCs for the problem behavior in question. Proximal drivers can include both antecedents and consequences of the problem behavior, so long as they occur proximally to the problem behavior. By proximal, a good rule of thumb is to think in terms of minutes or tens of minutes. Anything more distant would fall into the distal driver category discussed shortly.

Step 3. Contextual/Situational Information Gathering (or Determining the Establishing Operations)

Although contextual and situational influences are conceptually separate from drivers, many learning about FA for the first time have some trouble seeing how they differ from antecedents. Thus a first goal will be to disentangle them. Essentially, establishing operations are situational or contextual conditions that modify the targeted behavior. These conditions can be grouped into three categories: (1) physical (the surroundings), (2) social (who is around and what are they doing), and (3) medical/biological (what is happening in the body of the client). If antecedents are triggers, then establishing operations can be thought of as factors that increase or decrease sensitivity to that trigger. In research, these variables are sometimes called moderators because they moderate (or influence) the effect of another variable but are not viewed as causal. Drivers, on the other hand, are conceptualized as causally linked to the problem behavior.

Consider the example of a frazzled mother driving her three children home from a long weekend visit with their grandparents. Although things are initially quiet in the backseat, soon a squabble erupts. Imagine that squabbles serve as an antecedent for the mother's yelling at the children to stop. That is, when the kids squabble, the mother tends to yell. In therapy, further questions yield the fact that the yelling actually "works" because the squabbling generally stops for a time. Thus, after careful assessment, the therapist has accumulated solid data on the relevant antecedents and consequences related to the yelling behavior. Establishing operations that may affect such a situation could be physical (imagine the car's air conditioning is not working and it's summer), social (she is alone with her kids—perhaps she yells less when her partner or others are in the car), and medical/biological (she is hungry and has a headache).

Identifying establishing operations can be very helpful in assessing a problem because some of the "operations" can be foci for intervention. For example, keeping children well fed and well rested goes a long way toward reducing problematic behavior in the children (and in parents!). Similarly, knowing that loud music and having a lot of activity around makes it difficult for a child to complete his homework offers an easy first solution for the problem of homework completion. It is also worth noting that for some children, medical conditions can be important but overlooked establishing operations because many medical conditions affect psychological and emotional functioning. Thus it is often wise to discuss a child's medical history for a full understanding of the clinical situation.

Step 4. Distal Driver Nomination

In addition to proximal drivers and establishing operations, a good functional analysis also includes adequate consideration of historical variables, also known as distal drivers, that may influence the current problematic behavior (Henggeler et al., 2009). Discussion of distal drivers creates a good opportunity to dispel a myth that has developed about CBT—namely, that CBT therapists do not afford much time or credence to the importance of history, including clients' early childhood experiences. On the contrary, CBT therapists are avid historians, largely because of their understanding of how learning occurs. However, often CBT therapists focus on proximal factors (rather than distal factors) because they are ongoing, observable, and potentially malleable. Distal factors, unlike proximal factors, are rarely observable or malleable. For example, consider the adult client who reports a history of childhood emotional abuse. Although a CBT therapist will certainly consider that information in making a case conceptualization, the therapist also recognizes that she cannot change the client's history, only the client's present (and future). Thus the therapist will focus on the present and proximal drivers. However, because history often intrudes into the present through thoughts and memories—and thoughts and memories are potentially observable and malleable—history also can become part of the present focus of therapy.

There are numerous distal drivers to consider. Temperamental factors are a good example of a potential distal driver (although one could alternatively conceptualize temperament as an establishing operation). For example, some children have inhibited temperaments and are more likely to become anxious and engage in avoidance behaviors when confronted with novelty. In contrast, other children have stimulus-seeking temperaments that incline them to look for novelty and exciting experiences. Although the latter can have upsides, it can also lead to the child getting into dangerous situations or getting into trouble. Conceptualizing temperament as a distal driver underscores the point that a distal driver is not usually something that can change.

Another potential distal driver is any one of the client's past experiences, including how she was parented, her specific educational experiences (positive or negative), developmental experiences, abuse or trauma, or other negative or positive experiences. What differentiates a distal driver from a proximal one is that stimuli associated with the distal driver are no longer present, although they may be experienced (one assumes) internally, either through memories or thoughts.

As a simple example, consider a child who responds extremely negatively to touch, pulling away and looking angrily at the person who touched him. The therapist might hypothesize past maltreatment as a distal driver. But what might the proximal drivers be? To identify those, the therapist must consider the specific situation in which the client is touched. In this example, imagine that the child's reaction causes the "toucher" to cease the touching behavior and thus end the child's unpleasant feelings. Hence, negative reinforcement is present for both the "toucher" and the child. For the child, his extreme reaction to the touch led to a decrease in bad feelings; thus he will likely repeat those actions.

Another proximal driver in this case could be cognitive, like a thought or series of thoughts about touching. For example, the child may think to himself that all (or most) touching is malevolent in intent (researchers have referred to this as hostile attributional bias, whereby a person assumes hostile intent from others). Or he may simply experience touching as physically uncomfortable and thus may have a cascade of thoughts related to making the unpleasant feeling go away. He may even have thoughts relevant to the past maltreatment (i.e., "This feels like that time with Tom").

The example raises an important point about distal drivers that will serve as a conclusion to the section. Whereas it is true that distal drivers are by definition events "in the past," it is also true that many of them are "alive and well" in the present thanks to the fact that human beings are blessed with the ability to remember and re-experience past events. Some therapists applying FA for the first time are frustrated by what they perceive as the lack of prominence afforded to past events; however, with experience one can see that the past often intrudes into the present. Furthermore, it is not the past itself that intrudes, but rather a reproduction of the past, and usually an imperfect reproduction insofar as it contains distortions and misremembered aspects. Unlike the past event itself, the reproduction is malleable and thus is good fodder for the practitioner of FA.

APPLICATION OF FUNCTIONAL ANALYSES: TWO CASE STUDIES

To conclude the chapter, I describe two cases in some detail. For each, the FA model will be demonstrated step by step. Consistent with the focus of the book, the cases both warrant emotion-informed interventions. The focus here is on the initial case conceptualization; the next chapter addresses treatment selection for the cases presented here. All case material in this book has been altered to maximally protect the identity of clients. In some instances, a case described in the book is an amalgam of multiple cases.

Case 1: Chad

Chad is stocky 9-year-old boy who comes from a two-parent family; he is an only child. His parents brought him in for treatment for moderate behavior problems at home and school. For example, he regularly teases other kids at school and behaves defiantly at home, refusing to comply with rules and throwing frequent tantrums in response to limit setting. Although his teachers and the guidance counselor have suggested that Chad may have ADHD, there is no history of that diagnosis and no previous treatment of any kind. There is also no apparent precipitant to the current behavior. Chad has "always" acted like this. However, with each year it has "gotten a little worse." Now that the school has intervened by urging the parents to have Chad evaluated for services, the parents are taking some action.

The process of arranging the initial meeting reveals variable motivation to participate in treatment among the three family members and suggests the possibility that the family is somewhat disengaged. The father appears to have little time for his family; he did not attend either of the two scheduled intake appointments, and the therapist was not able to arrange a phone meeting despite repeated efforts. During the first two sessions, the mother and child choose to sit in separate armchairs, despite the possibility of sharing a large couch. They are observed to interact in a rather perfunctory manner. It is always hard to know how much a role anxiety plays when family members act stiffly in formal situations like an evaluation meeting. Still, the therapist notes the physical distance between mother and son as well as the lack of emotional expression.

The mother, an unassertive and highly anxious woman in her late 30s, provides descriptions of the situation that suggest ambivalence about the problems. Although she would like Chad's misbehavior to decrease, she feels badly when her son is not happy. For example, she suggests, through her descriptions, that she may be guilty of reinforcing misbehavior through either failing to follow through with punishments or by directly attending to Chad when he is having a tantrum. During the meeting, she also reinforces Chad when he whines about being thirsty by giving him a dollar for the soda machine. She also hints at guilt that her husband is not around more to be with Chad, noting that she thinks Chad "needs a connection with his dad."

Discussion of the typical problems in the home reveals the following set of transactions. Chad requests something like additional TV time and his mother's first response is "No." Chad escalates his requests from arguing to angry shouting and even door slamming. In most instances, the mother capitulates, afterward retreating to her own room in frustration. According to the mother's report, Chad uses a similar *persistence* strategy at school to get his way. A phone call with his homeroom teacher confirms this, with the additional finding that he bullies other children to get his way, engaging in name calling and, sometimes, physical intimidation.

A review of his school records and an individual meeting with Chad helps the therapist to learn more about this young man. Although Chad comes across as angry in his verbalizations, the therapist hypothesizes that Chad actually is sad and anxious. For example, he uses angry words in blaming his parents and teachers for having too many rules, yet his facial expressions seem sad. When asked in a number of ways how he feels about the various problem situations at home and school, the therapist notes the poverty of Chad's descriptions. He uses the words "bad" and "ticked-off" almost exclusively. When asked about goals, he says he wants to get his mom and the teachers off his back, but he also admits he would like to get into less trouble and even assents to a suggestion that he would like to get along better with his peers.

The evaluation also included the collection of a variety of psychometric measures from Chad, his mother, and his teacher. Measures were sent home for the father to complete, but he opted not to do so. After scoring the measures, the therapist notes that although there are expectable high scores on measures capturing behavior problems, the teacher also endorses a relatively high degree of depressive symptoms. Not surprisingly, Chad endorses very few symptoms, and all of his self-reported scores are within normal limits. Overall, the evaluation suggests a diagnosis of oppositional defiant disorder with a rule-out for mood disorder not otherwise specified (NOS). Although the school had speculated that Chad has ADHD, the evaluation does not support that diagnosis, although the inattentive subtype cannot be ruled out definitively without additional assessment.

With the details available at this point, the therapist can use the steps of functional analysis steps to identify (1) problems, (2) proximal drivers, (3) contextual factors, (4) distal drivers, and finally (5) possible interventions. In this chapter, the focus is on the first four of these steps. In Chapter 5, Chad's case, as well as Brittney's, which follows, are reprised to complete the final step: intervention selection.

Step 1. Identify the Problems

The first step is to create a list of problems based on what was known so far; Figure 4.1 summarizes the three problems identified.

The first two problems definitely meet the criteria of *good* problem definitions described earlier in that each is (1) simple, (2) specific and observable, and (3) potentially changeable. The third problem is the most speculative, given the greater difficulty involved in observing Chad's emotional awareness and understanding. The mother reported (and to some extent, so did Chad) that when he is "bothered," his go-to coping skill is aggression, either verbal or physical. That aggression leads to problems 1 and 2. What is not clear is exactly what the "bothered" feeling is like for Chad. This lack of clarity suggests the possibility of an emotion-related deficit—that is, Chad's lack of knowledge about what he is feeling may be a problem worth addressing. Although the therapist can work with the family to change antecedents and consequences, without knowing what is happening inside Chad—what meaning he is making of the situations—the risk for future difficulties remains if he does not learn to identify and regulate his own emotions. Hence, the third problem, although speculative and difficult to observe without Chad's help, remains an important hypothesized problem to address.

Problems	1. Argues and throws tantrums to get his way (at home)	2. Bullies and intimidates to get his way (at school)	3. Does not understand or will not express his internal emotional state
Proximal drivers (antecedents)			
Proximal drivers (consequences)			
Contextual/ situational factors			
Distal drivers			

FIGURE 4.1. Chad's functional analysis: Problems.

Step 2. Identify the Proximal Drivers

After settling on the problems, the therapist can proceed to Step 2: identifying proximal drivers. As the reader will recall, there are two categories to consider here: antecedents, or those events that occur before the problem behavior, and consequences, or those events that occur after the problem behavior.

Antecedents

Chad, like many children, is triggered when he does not get his way; in other words, when his will is thwarted in some way, or his desires are blocked, he becomes upset and often copes in maladjusted ways. This antecedent was deemed relevant for the first two problems. A more speculative antecedent for problems 1 and 2 may be Chad's internal conversation. Here, possibilities abound. Perhaps he is postulating about the stupidity of others? Or how others should meet his needs? Or that force is the only way to get those needs met? Alternatively, he may have more sensitive thoughts like "Succeeding this way makes me a bad person," or "Why don't people like me or listen to me unless I am causing a fuss?" Of course, these are only speculations. However, Chad has, over time, developed a set of beliefs about these situations, and the thoughts themselves may be antecedents to the behaviors. For example, if his mother says no to Chad and he thinks, "She is wrong—she will change her mind," and then he proceeds to argue, Chad's thought that his mother will change her mind is an antecedent to his arguing behavior.

Another potentially relevant, yet also speculative, antecedent for problem 2 may be Chad's perception of threat from peers. He may be a child who sees threats and chooses to respond quickly to reduce those threats, perhaps in response to a belief that aggression will be an effective and/or appropriate strategy in such cases.

Two antecedent drivers are noted for problem 3. First, the therapist hypothesizes that Chad is more likely to be befuddled by his emotions when those emotions are intense. Struggling with strong emotions is common, but for children like Chad who may be ill-equipped to understand and deal with any emotions, the problem is magnified. A second possible driver is Chad's reluctance to discuss his feelings. As he experiences strong emotions throughout the day, his failure to share those emotions as a means of coping may predispose him to become more dysregulated as a day wears on. As noted earlier, the drivers for problem 3 are necessarily more tentative than the drivers of the other problems given the lack of observability of Chad's internal emotional state.

Consequences

Inconsistent parenting is an obvious contributor to both problems 1 and 2. Chad's mother regularly reinforces Chad's problem behaviors at home (i.e., pushing limits, arguing, and even slamming the door to his room) and does not punish him for his reported misbehavior at school. Chad's bullying of other children at school, while earning him some punishment, has also yielded positive results: he is getting his way in many social situations and also earning the respect, if not the affection, of his peers. Concerning problem 3, the therapist hypothesizes that Chad's parents do not use these emotionally charged situations as opportunities to teach Chad how to identify and deal with his emotions, thereby sustaining Chad's apparent lack of emotional knowledge. Figure 4.2 summarizes these findings and hypotheses.

Step 3. Gather Situational and Contextual Information (or Identify Establishing Operations)

As noted earlier, establishing operations fall into three categories: physical, social, and medical/biological. In Chad's case, there is one prominent social context variable related to his family: Chad's misbehavior is much more common when he is alone with his mother than when he is alone with his father or when both parents are present. Regarding the school-related problem, the therapist's impression was that Chad is more likely to have trouble when there were a lot of peers around rather than just a few. In other words, he is less likely to bully others in a small group. The therapist also noted a medical/biological factor: the possible diagnosis of ADHD, inattentive type, which could influence all three problem areas. No other contextual influences were noted. Figure 4.3 adds the contextual/situational factors hypothesized for Chad.

Step 4. Identify Distal Drivers

Distal drivers are historical variables that may influence the current situation. No obvious past trauma or other highly negative experience was apparent. However, there did appear to be a history of limited family emotion socialization that no doubt would have influenced problem 3. Nothing in Chad's history suggested reason to speculate about other distal drivers at this point. Figure 4.4 summarizes the findings to this point.

At this point, the therapist's next steps would be treatment selection and sequencing, which are covered in the next chapter. Chad's treatment plan will be discussed there in detail. Next, a second case is presented to provide an additional example of the application of FA.

Case 2: Brittney

Brittney is a 14-year-old girl living with her mother and younger brother (age 9). The primary complaint bringing the family to the clinic was that Brittney gets really "freaked out" over peer relationships, at times spending days in her room upset. The therapist learned, for example, that Brittney had heard a few boys were saying mean things about one of her friends. She was so upset about the event that she

Problems	1. Argues and throws tantrums to get his way (at home)	2. Bullies and intimidates to get his way (at school)	3. Does not understand or will not express his internal emotional state
Proximal drivers (antecedents)	**Desires blocked** **Thoughts or beliefs (e.g., about the effectiveness of force or arguing, about his not being good at tough situations)**	**Desires blocked** **Thoughts or beliefs (e.g., about the effectiveness of force or arguing, about his not being good at tough situations)** **Threatened by a peer**	**Experiences intense emotion** **Not having discussed tough experiences from the day**
Proximal drivers (consequences)	**Parental reinforcement of misbehavior** **Lack of parental punishment of misbehavior**	**Peer reinforcement of misbehavior** **Lack of parental punishment of misbehavior**	**Lack of parental teaching on emotion**
Contextual/ situational factors			
Distal drivers			

FIGURE 4.2. Chad's functional analysis: Proximal drivers.

Problems	1. Argues and throws tantrums to get his way (at home)	2. Bullies and intimidates to get his way (at school)	3. Does not understand or will not express his internal emotional state
Proximal drivers (antecedents)	Desires blocked Thoughts or beliefs (e.g., about the effectiveness of force or arguing, about his not being good at tough situations)	Desires blocked Thoughts or beliefs (e.g., about the effectiveness of force or arguing, about his not being good at tough situations) Threatened by a peer	Experiences intense emotion Not having discussed tough experiences from the day
Proximal drivers (consequences)	Parental reinforcement of misbehavior Lack of parental punishment of misbehavior	Peer reinforcement of misbehavior Lack of parental punishment of misbehavior	Lack of parental teaching on emotion
Contextual/ situational factors	**When father is not present** **Diagnosis of ADHD**	**When around a large number of peers** **Diagnosis of ADHD**	**Diagnosis of ADHD**
Distal drivers			

FIGURE 4.3. Chad's functional analysis: Contextual/situational factors.

Problems	1. Argues and throws tantrums to get his way (at home)	2. Bullies and intimidates to get his way (at school)	3. Does not understand or will not express his internal emotional state
Proximal drivers (antecedents)	Desires blocked Thoughts or beliefs (e.g., about the effectiveness of force or arguing, about his not being good at tough situations)	Desires blocked Thoughts or beliefs (e.g., about the effectiveness of force or arguing, about his not being good at tough situations) Threatened by a peer	Experiences intense emotion Not having discussed tough experiences from the day
Proximal drivers (consequences)	Parental reinforcement of misbehavior Lack of parental punishment of misbehavior	Peer reinforcement of misbehavior Lack of parental punishment of misbehavior	Lack of parental teaching on emotion
Contextual/ situational factors	When father is not present Diagnosis of ADHD	When around a large number of peers Diagnosis of ADHD	Diagnosis of ADHD
Distal drivers			**Poor family emotion socialization**

FIGURE 4.4. Chad's functional analysis: Distal drivers.

spent 2 days alone in her room, alternately crying and writing in her journal. She also experienced extreme upset when a close friend, Todd, was feeling down. The mother noted that Todd had always seemed like a really depressed young man, and the mother knew from Brittney that he engaged in self-injurious behaviors. Brittney and Todd talked on the phone a lot, especially at night. In the weeks leading up to the referral for treatment, Brittney had become more withdrawn, spending most of her time alone or on the phone with Todd. In addition, the mother described instances where Brittney erupted in anger at peers and her family, even cursing out her best female friends at school. After these episodes, the mother noted that Brittney was even more withdrawn.

Data gathered during intake meetings indicated that Brittney was experiencing significant depression and anxiety. In intake meetings, she appeared depressed: her eyes were downcast, she appeared tired, her voice tone was flat, and her speech content focused on the negative. In the meetings and on a set of standardized measures, Brittney and her mother (separately) reported that Brittney was exhibiting a number of DSM-IV symptoms of depression (e.g., depressed mood, anhedonia, trouble sleeping, excessive guilt, poor appetite). They also reported many anxiety symptoms, most of which were consistent with the DSM-IV categories of generalized anxiety disorder (e.g., she worries a lot about others' well-being, as well as other topics like her schoolwork) and social phobia (e.g., she is afraid that others will reject her, she avoids some social situations at school). Several areas of strength emerged as well: Brittney was articulate and thoughtful; the mother was engaged and concerned, though busy; and Brittney had a social support network among her peers, albeit threatened by some of her angry outbursts.

Step 1. Identify the Problems

The problems here started off murky and broad rather than simple, specific, and changeable. In the first session, Brittney described herself as a cheerful and good friend. She said she liked helping others with their problems and noted that her friends often say she is a good listener. She even confided with a wink that she might like to have a job as a therapist one day. However, her presentation in therapy was not always cheerful. In one session, Brittney was unusually quiet and would only talk about how upsetting it had been for her to hear about her friend Todd's current problems. At times like this, inquiries for details about her cognitive or emotional state would yield very little. Asking the mother for more details ended in disappointment—she was not able to add much more to the description of the situation.

In short, although Brittney behaved like someone who was depressed (withdrawn, crying) and anxious (avoiding specific social interactions, worrying excessively about others), the assessment had many gaps. It's not uncommon to lack details at the start of a case, which makes Brittney's case a good example of how to use FA in less than ideal circumstances. Here, the therapist might settle on three problems: high levels of depressed mood, overfocus on negative events (rumination), and social isolation (see Figure 4.5).

Step 2. Identify the Proximal Drivers

Antecedents

Brittney's episodes of rumination and isolation (problems 2 and 3) tend to be triggered by adverse peer events. Sometimes these events involve her directly (e.g., being teased by a peer), but more often she is merely observing a difficult situation happening to another. Brittney and her mother both gave numerous accounts of times when a friend of Brittney's was upset or "wronged" that ended with Brittney spending time ruminating alone or with the friend and then feeling upset for long periods. Relatedly, and relevant for problems 1 and 2, the distress of others was highly contagious for Brittney. Readers can recall the section on empathy in Chapter 2. Brittney's response to others' pain appears at first to be strongly empathic, but it is more accurately described as a reaction of personal distress. That is, she feels the pain of others so strongly that she has a hard time separating from "feeling with" another person in order to offer help.

Another antecedent driver, while more tentatively offered than the first, is Brittney's expectations of others' responses to her: she guesses that others are going to perceive her negatively. Brittney has described many of her peers in unfavorable ways, stating that they are often untrustworthy and cruel. Although there is some evidence to back her up, she also appears to have a general expectation that she will be treated unkindly. Even within her circle, she reports fears that her friends secretly dislike her. The therapist could hypothesize that these beliefs serve an antecedent role in driving all three of Brittney's identified problems.

Consequences

Brittney appears to cope with upsetting stimuli through continued direct exposure to the upsetting stimuli (e.g., long phone calls with Todd) and indirect exposure through rumination (e.g., thinking about what others said or did to her or her friends). The first of these strategies can often be a helpful method; social support is an important and effective coping strategy for many people. However, in Brittney's case, the social support was actually reinforcing her rumination on negative events and expectations, thereby contributing to her depressed mood. In short, she was obtaining positive attention from her peers for having and dwelling on upsetting events (and perceptions).

If a possible antecedent to Brittney's behavior is her negative expectations about others, a consequence of her rumination and isolation could be that those negative beliefs about others are strengthened. The therapist observed that Brittney does not often seek much (or any) information that might contradict her beliefs

Problems	1. High levels of depressed mood	2. Overfocus on negative events (rumination)	3. Social isolation
Proximal drivers (antecedents)			
Proximal drivers (consequences)			
Contextual/ situational factors			
Distal drivers			

FIGURE 4.5. Brittney's functional analysis: Problems.

about others, preferring instead to dwell on the reasons why her beliefs were justified. Some readers may recall this phenomenon from their introductory psychology
class: a self-fulfilling prophecy.

A third and related consequence is most directly related to Brittney's isolation
and rumination. Because she does not attempt to make friends outside of her small
circle and spends most of her time alone, she is not exposed to new events, some
of which might provide "contrary" evidence. For example, she has little firsthand
evidence to support her guess that others do not like her or her friends. Perhaps
some of her peers do find her odd at times, but it's just as likely that some peers find
her interesting or "friend-worthy." In short, a consequence of remaining isolated is
that Brittney does not have the opportunity to learn anything new about her social
world; instead she "learns" what she already "knows" and believes. Figure 4.6 summarizes these findings and hypotheses.

Step 3. Gather Situational and Contextual Information
(or Identify Establishing Operations)

Recall that Brittney is, at 14, in early adolescence; normal developmental processes
are moving her away from the sphere of the home and family toward her peers.
Consider, too, that the time she shares with her family has already been limited
for a number of reasons. First, she lives in a single-parent home, and her mother
has a demanding work schedule (one full-time job during the week and a part-
time job on the weekend). Second, when her mother is around she has a number
of household tasks to attend to in addition to spending time with her two children.
Third, the mother has been lulled into a false security due to her son's apparent self-
sufficiency and Brittney's apparent desire for autonomy. Finally, it is relevant to note
that Brittney's father has been absent since shortly after the divorce and currently
lives in a different state. Overall, the therapist could describe the context here as
one of relative parental neglect, although not in the formal (and reportable) sense.
Brittney lacks the listening ear and timely advice from a trusted adult. During the
initial interview, the mother admitted that she had grown to think of Brittney as
self-maintaining and that Brittney's recent increased isolation and depressed behaviors had been a wake-up call to the gravity of the situation. This establishing operation (the relative absence of parental support/guidance) may contribute to all three
of her problems.

Two additional contextual factors should be considered. First, Brittney was
clearly vulnerable to the distress of others. Rather than responding in an empathic
and instrumentally helpful manner, Brittney appeared to be disproportionately
upset by others' distress and lacking in the coping skills to help herself or the other
person. History from the mother indicated Brittney has always been susceptible to
the feelings of others. Indeed, during the divorce, when Brittney was 5, the mother
recalled noticing that Brittney was often upset when she herself was upset. Thus
she had a high sensitivity to interpersonally stressful situations, a temperamental

Problems	1. High levels of depressed mood	2. Overfocus on negative events (rumination)	3. Social isolation
Proximal drivers (antecedents)	Others' distress Expects others to view her negatively	Adverse peer events Others' distress Expects others to view her negatively	Adverse peer events Expects others to view her negatively
Proximal drivers (consequences)	"Rewarded" by peers for problems	"Rewarded" by peers for problems Negative thoughts are "rewarded" Lack of exposure to "contrary" evidence	Negative thoughts are "rewarded" Lack of exposure to "contrary" evidence
Contextual/ situational factors			
Distal drivers			

FIGURE 4.6. Brittney's functional analysis: Proximal drivers.

"context" that may be contributing to all three of her problems. Brittney's maternal family's history of depression (Brittney's maternal grandmother and two of her maternal aunts had all suffered from depression) may also contribute to all three problems. Figure 4.7 summarizes the findings to this point.

Step 4. Identify Distal Drivers

Consideration of distal factors starts with the fact that there was a family history of depression. Although there may have been a genetic predisposition, the "nurture" side of the equation seems a possible contributor to Brittney's current difficulties. Brittney's mother grew up with a depressed mother and two depressed sisters herself. Might Brittney's mother have opted to steer clear of these three depressed women as a way to cope, thereby modeling social isolation? And how might that early coping have affected her reaction to Brittney when she first demonstrated signs of depression? Obviously, to confirm such hypotheses, the therapist would need to learn more about the mother's reactions to Brittney's depression.

Another potential and likely distal factor was the fact that Brittney's parents were divorced when she was 5. The divorce was described as a contentious one that, although not violent, was full of verbal rancor between the parents, often not well modulated in the presence of the children. In addition, the mother was regularly distressed and unable to shield her 5-year-old daughter from witnessing her weeping or raging on the phone to friends. The ramifications for the divorce were several, including the absence of a father figure for Brittney, the lack of additional adult support in the home, and the occurrence early in development of an upsetting relational disruption. One might hypothesize that some or even many of Brittney's current relational difficulties may be echoes of the divorce experience. Indeed, seeds for some of Brittney's current beliefs may have been planted during this important experience. Thus the distal driver of the divorce may contribute to all three problem areas (see Figure 4.8).

Once the initial conceptualization is complete, the therapist's next step would be to identify interventions to address the contributing factors to the problems described here, a task left to the next chapter.

CONCLUSION

As stated at the outset, FA is a useful approach for clinical work, both for children who will benefit from emotion-informed interventions and for other children as well. FA is such a potent tool because it helps therapists flexibly address multiple client problems and provides a blueprint for how to conceptualize a case and build a treatment plan that is individualized for each client. The next chapter focuses on how to use FA as a means to formulate treatment plans that test the validity of the case conceptualization by targeting drivers.

Problems	1. High levels of depressed mood	2. Overfocus on negative events (rumination)	3. Social isolation
Proximal drivers (antecedents)	Others' distress Expects others to view her negatively	Adverse peer events Others' distress Expects others to view her negatively	Adverse peer events Expects others to view her negatively
Proximal drivers (consequences)	"Rewarded" by peers for problems	"Rewarded" by peers for problems Negative thoughts are "rewarded" Lack of exposure to "contrary" evidence	 Negative thoughts are "rewarded" Lack of exposure to "contrary" evidence
Contextual/ situational factors	**Relative absence of adult support** **Temperamental vulnerability to others' distress** **Predisposition to depression**	**Relative absence of adult support** **Temperamental vulnerability to others' distress** **Predisposition to depression**	**Relative absence of adult support** **Temperamental vulnerability to others' distress** **Predisposition to depression**
Distal drivers			

FIGURE 4.7. Brittney's functional analysis: Contextual/situational factors added.

Problems	1. High levels of depressed mood	2. Overfocus on negative events (rumination)	3. Social isolation
Proximal drivers (antecedents)	Others' distress Expects others to view her negatively	Adverse peer events Others' distress Expects others to view her negatively	Adverse peer events Expects others to view her negatively
Proximal drivers (consequences)	"Rewarded" by peers for problems	"Rewarded" by peers for problems Negative thoughts are "rewarded" Lack of exposure to "contrary" evidence	Negative thoughts are "rewarded" Lack of exposure to "contrary" evidence
Contextual/ situational factors	Relative absence of adult support Temperamental vulnerability to others' distress Predisposition to depression	Relative absence of adult support Temperamental vulnerability to others' distress Predisposition to depression	Relative absence of adult support Temperamental vulnerability to others' distress Predisposition to depression
Distal drivers	**Parents' divorce**	**Parents' divorce**	**Mother's experience in a depressed family** **Parents' divorce**

FIGURE 4.8. Brittney's functional analysis: Distal drivers.

FUNCTIONAL ANALYSIS RESOURCES

Freeman, K. A., & Miller, C. A. (2002). Behavioral case conceptualization for children and adolescents. In M Hersen (Ed.), *Clinical behavior therapy: Adults and children* (pp. 239–255). New York: Wiley.

Henggeler, S. W., Schoenwald, S. K., Borduin, C. M., Rowland, M. D., & Cunningham, P. B. (2009). *Multisystemic therapy for antisocial behavior in children and adolescents* (2nd ed.). New York: Guilford Press.

Persons, J. B. (2008). *The case formulation approach to cognitive-behavior therapy.* New York: Guilford Press.

CHAPTER 5

Treatment Planning

Combining Functional Analysis and Modularity

This chapter introduces the treatment concept of modularity, which, together with functional analysis, drives the remaining content of the book. The idea of modularity is not a new one, and it has been applied in a variety of fields, from building construction and automobiles to home furniture and children's toys. Briefly, modular design involves using individual parts that can function independently but that can also be combined (generally in any order) without loss of information and without preconditions. The familiar Lego bricks are largely modular. Each brick is a separate and stand-alone item, and bricks can be combined in a variety of ways to form many different objects. For instance, one can use Lego bricks to make a car, a helicopter, or a boat (or a heli-boat-car!). For more information on modularity, the interested reader can see the article by Chorpita, Daleiden, and Weisz (2005). This approach can be contrasted with what are called *integral* designs, in which the parts are interdependent and thus not decomposable.

This chapter covers modularity as a treatment method; explains the format of the modules included in this book; discusses the transition from conceptualization to treatment planning using functional analysis; and, finally, revisits the cases of Chad and Brittney, introduced in Chapter 4, to illustrate how functional analysis can serve as a guide to treatment planning.

MODULARITY

Modularity involves the creation or identification of individual parts called modules that can be used to create something (e.g., a couch, a treatment plan). Specific to therapy, treatment modules are independent insofar as they are stand-alone products; they do not need other modules to function as designed. This means that each module must contain *all* the information required to accomplish its goals without reference to other modules. If using a truly modular treatment, a therapist can pick up any module and use it at any point in therapy with a client, regardless of what has come before or after. Such a level of flexibility has great strengths for busy clinicians with caseloads full of multiproblem clients. If the primary problem shifts, the ability of modular approaches to turn on a dime is a great advantage.

When modules are combined, though, other benefits of modular design arise. There is often a default ordering of a set of treatment modules for a particular problem. For example, consider anxiety disorders in children. Chorpita (2007) suggests a default order as follows: Engagement module, Fear Ladder module, Psychoeducation module, Exposure module, and Maintenance module. Others have suggested alternative defaults (e.g., Kendall, Hudson, Gosch, Flannery-Schroeder, & Suveg, 2008). However, because modules are designed to fit together regardless of the order, a therapist can create his or her own order, guided by case-specific data.

Modularity is different from *business as usual*. One reason for this difference is that it avoids the so-called *multiple manual problem*. It is important to know that few developers of treatment manuals originally viewed the manuals as the ultimate goal. Instead, the idea was to use a manual as a method to clearly define the treatment for research purposes. However, as treatment manuals proliferated and the evidence-based treatment movement became larger and more vocal, manuals were seen as terrific vehicles for dissemination of treatment programs. If they worked in the research studies, why not just train therapists to use them in practice?

Scientists and practitioners have generated a host of reasons to be cautious in applying manuals *as-is* across an array of settings in which their use has not been tested. Clients in research studies may (and apparently do) differ from clients seen in other settings, like public mental health clinics. There are data suggesting that research study clients have fewer comorbid problems and have greater demographic advantages (e.g., higher incomes, more stable family lives, less stress) compared to clients in public mental health clinics (e.g., Ehrenreich et al., 2011; Southam-Gerow, Chorpita, Miller, & Gleacher, 2008; Southam-Gerow, Weisz, & Kendall, 2003). In addition, therapists in research studies carry a small caseload, sometimes as low as four or five cases, with intensive supervision often provided by the treatment developer. In contrast, many clinicians in community settings carry 20 or more cases and have perhaps an hour of weekly supervision (Weisz, Southam-Gerow, Gordis, & Connor-Smith, 2003). Finally, research studies often rely on grant funds and only rarely occur in clinics where client fees and insurance payments are needed to pay operating expenses. These and other differences have suggested a need to consider adaptations necessary to use these programs in contexts beyond research studies.

A thorough review of the potential limitations of evidence-based treatment manuals is outside of the scope of this book, and the interested reader can consult a number of sources for further information (Schoenwald & Hoagwood, 2001;

Southam-Gerow, Rodriguez, Chorpita, & Daleiden, in press; Weisz et al., 2003). Here, it is enough to say that manuals are usually designed for a single focal problem, like anxiety, depression, or oppositional defiant disorder. A single-problem approach may be appropriate for some clients (or many—the applicability is an empirical question). However, for those clients with multiple problems, the specter of the multiple-manual problem looms.

Consider an analogous situation from the medical world. Imagine a person with a cold. Her cold has many symptoms, including a cough, runny nose, and a headache. The good news is that there are medicines for each of those symptoms, and even better, there are cold medicines that can treat all of her symptoms at the same time. Now imagine that in addition to her cold, she is also experiencing heartburn. Of course, there is a medicine for that, too. Now imagine she also happens to have athlete's foot. Yes, there is medicine for that, too. With medicine, it can be relatively simple to combine therapies, although drug interactions can be complex. But the mechanics of the treatment are usually straightforward: the patient swallows a dose of the cold medicine, chews two antacid tablets, and applies an antifungal cream to her feet. In total, the treatment session for all three problems might take her 1 minute.

However, in the realm of psychological treatments, things can be much more complicated, even for nonemergency problems. To keep it simple, imagine a child client with two different problems. How should you treat him, given that each treatment manual can take 12 or more sessions to complete? Should you use two manuals simultaneously? Or would treatment proceed serially—that is, first he gets treatment A and then treatment B? Either approach has problems. Simultaneous treatment assumes that a client has 2 hours a week to dedicate to treatment and that the client can work in parallel fashion through both treatments. Serial treatment assumes that the therapist can identify which manual should go first and that the client has at least 24 weeks to dedicate to treatment. Both approaches assume the therapist is an expert on both manuals. As the number of client problems goes up, the multiple-manual problem only becomes more pronounced.

Using a modular treatment is one way to avoid the multiple-manual problem while retaining the flexibility necessary to address cases with multiple presenting problems. The modular approach allows a clinician to build a treatment plan one module at a time, knowing that with a change in focus (e.g., new problem emerges, different primary problem becomes clear, conceptualization of case shifts to prioritize different primary drivers), different modules can be used without disrupting the flow of treatment by introducing a new manual.

IDENTIFYING TREATMENT STRATEGIES

Initial efforts to identify empirically supported treatments focused on (1) creating criteria for judging the evidence for a treatment, (2) reviewing the literature, and

(3) scoring treatments using the criteria established (e.g., Chambless et al., 1996). As most readers know, the effort resulted in lists of treatments with titles such as "empirically supported treatments," "empirically validated treatments," "evidence-based treatments," "evidence-based practices," and even "promising practices." Although this chapter describes an approach that arguably improves on this framework, the progress generated by the work of the pioneers of evidence-based treatments cannot be overstated.

And yet there are a number of limitations to the method of identifying treatments described above. These include (1) lack of consensus on what the criteria should be, leading to a plethora of lists; (2) failure to address the issue of "expiration" (how old is too old for a study to support a treatment?); and (3) focus limited to published studies, despite the possibility that good treatments occur outside of the realm of science.

In addition, two problems are particularly germane to modularity. First is the multiple manual problem described above. Second is what Chorpita and Daleiden (2009) has called the "crowded-cell" problem. To understand this problem, imagine a set of boxes or cells, each representing a problem area like anxiety. For some problems, many different treatment programs "crowd" the cell. This may seem like good news—there are many options! However, crowded cells can make it difficult for a therapist to select a treatment program for a client, especially if the evidence is largely the same for each option. These potential pitfalls in treatment identification have led some researchers to offer new and creative ways to build on and improve the process of evidence-based treatment identification.

Practice Element Distillation

One such effort has been called practice element distillation (Chorpita & Daleiden, 2009). Recall the crowded-cell problem. The cell for child conduct problems contains a number of different treatment programs, although many of them could be broadly defined as "parent training" approaches. One solution would be to create a generic parent training program that captures all the elements found in the several different programs with an evidence base. An alternative solution, and the one utilized by this book, is to distill the various evidence-based programs down to their fundamental parts and use those parts to guide the new treatment approach.

So how does distillation work? Chorpita and Daleiden (2009) have outlined one method. The primary steps are familiar: search the literature and identify treatment programs with varying levels of empirical support. Here the approach distinguishes itself: identify the fundamental parts ("practice elements") of each program with empirical support. Practice elements can be viewed as the important principles or skills of a treatment program; examples for parent training include parent psychoeducation (i.e., teaching parents about the determinants of child behavior and misbehavior), rewards (i.e., working with parents to design and implement reward systems in their home), and time out (i.e., working with parents to implement the time-out procedure to punish child misbehavior). Once the practice elements have been identified, a stand-alone module can be created for each one. In other words, the practice elements are modularized. This process results in a library of discrete principles or skills to teach and practice with a client. The therapist can order the modules to fit the case rather than follow the order of a particular treatment program. Furthermore, because multiple programs are distilled, it is possible to address multiple problems. While it may be possible to treat multiple problems by creating a single large treatment program, the client may wonder, "Why do I have to sit through three meetings on X when the problem I really have is Y?" In short, the modular approach as realized through practice element distillation represents a promising approach to treatment, one for which evidence is accumulating (e.g., Chorpita, Taylor, Francis, Moffit, & Austin, 2004; Weisz et al., 2012).

THE STANDARD ELEMENTS OF A MODULE

Having described the defining characteristics of modularity, it is now time to turn to a description of what a module looks. For this book, the standards developed by Chorpita (2007) have been followed, although in a modified, briefer form. Each module in this book includes the following three sections.

1. *When to Use This Module.* This section offers a description for when the therapist might choose to use the module. For example, which problem areas do the module target?
2. *Objectives.* This section offers a brief synopsis of the goals of the module. There are generally three to five goals per module that serve as checklist for the more detailed procedures described in the third section. As such, they could be used as a reminder to a clinician who is already experienced with the module.
3. *Procedures.* The third section is the *main course* of each module. This consists of three subsections: (a) Overview, describing the session's objectives in more details; (b) Teach, detailing the session's main teaching points and illustrating those points with case examples; and (c) Practice, offering games and activities designed to reinforce the teaching points. For some procedures, there are no activities or games provided because some of the teaching points are straightforward or do not lend themselves to games. Some of the modules also have worksheets and handouts, available at the end of the applicable module.

Often in skill-based therapies, there is a tension between providing a rationale for a particular skill and teaching that skill didactically on one hand, and keeping the focus practice oriented (i.e., activity based) on the other hand. For most of the modules in the book, despite their emphasis on activities, providing the client with the rationale for focusing on a particular skill is warranted for a few reasons. First, the treatment is designed be as transparent as possible. The strategies presented here are not secret or magical. It is fair to assume that many clients will appreciate and gain from an approach that clearly details the strategies being used and the reasons for their use. Second, for some clients, knowing what the "point" is will help them better learn the skill. That is, if a client knows why he is learning about feelings (e.g., to help him get along better with others or to help him learn how to calm down when he is angry or stressed), he may feel more inclined to actively participate in the Practice sections of the meetings.

That said, in some cases providing a rationale may unnecessarily complicate the session if given too early or at all. For example, consider John, a socially anxious 16-year-old with symptoms of Asperger syndrome. As the therapist began to explain the rationale for treatment, John found a reason to query each aspect of the rationale, expressing doubt about the approach's effectiveness and lack of confidence in therapy. Rather than continuing to pursue her case for the approach rationally, the therapist opted to emphasize practice in meetings, and the treatment began to proceed somewhat more smoothly. For some clients, jumping right into the Practice section of the modules may be the best course.

Role Playing

Role playing is a common Practice technique used in many of the modules. Although some clients are eager to practice, many prefer to see what the therapist's expectation is first. Hence, therapists should be ready to model. *Coping modeling*, wherein the therapist provides an imperfect model of the behavior, is generally preferred to *mastery modeling*, wherein the therapist provides a perfect model. Obviously, clear demonstration of the relevant aspects of a particular behavior is important. The coping model should be thorough; however, it is also useful for a child to see that the practice is not perfect. An example of a role play from a session with Molly, an extremely socially anxious (nearly selectively mute at the start of treatment) 16-year-old. Here, after several sessions of behavioral exposures reducing the client's anxiety in interactions with the therapist and a few other adults, the therapist prepares Molly for future exposures to occur in public settings. In this excerpt, they are role-playing ordering at a restaurant.

THERAPIST: Okay, let's practice. You be the person at the fast-food restaurant taking my order, and I'll make an order. So, let's see, where would you stand if you worked there?

MOLLY: I don't know, at the cash register?

THERAPIST: Sounds right. Let's pretend the cash register is here, okay? So you stand there and I'll come up to you. Your job here will be to tell me how much my order costs.

[as customer] Hi. Um, I want . . . hmm . . . a chicken sandwich and . . . something to drink. Iced tea? No, a Sprite.

MOLLY: Um . . .

THERAPIST: Oh, right. What would that cost? Let's say $5.50?

MOLLY: Okay, $5.50.

THERAPIST: [as customer]: Okay. Here you go.
[as therapist] And scene. Okay, great job running the register! Let's talk about what you saw *me* do.

MOLLY: You ordered.

THERAPIST: Right. What did I say?

MOLLY: What you wanted. A sandwich and . . . a drink.

THERAPIST: Right—great! Is that what you think would happen?

MOLLY: Yeah, I guess. I might mess up.

THERAPIST: Did you notice if I messed up?

MOLLY: Um, no. You just said your order.

THERAPIST: Are you sure I didn't mess up? With my drink?

MOLLY: Oh, you changed your order.

THERAPIST: Am I allowed to do that?

MOLLY: I think so. I'm not sure.

[After further discussion . . .]

THERAPIST: Okay, so let's have you try it. You be the customer. I'll be here at the register. Do you remember what you're going to say?

MOLLY: Um, my order?

THERAPIST: Yup! Will it help to know exactly what you are going to order before you come up?

MOLLY: Probably.

THERAPIST: So what will you order?

MOLLY: How about what you did?

THERAPIST: Sounds great. What was that?

MOLLY: A chicken sandwich and a drink.

THERAPIST: What drink?

MOLLY: Sprite.

THERAPIST: I think you're ready. First, though, what is your anxiety rating? On a scale of 0 to 10, with 10 being super anxious about doing this.

MOLLY: Maybe a 4?

All of the exercises and experiences described in each module are culled from experiences and examples in my career as therapist and supervisor. However, readers are encouraged to be creative and riff on the sample exercises and activities described in the book to find their own ways to accomplish the objectives of the modules. In short, the examples here are meant as guides and not as prescriptions.

ADDITIONAL SESSION ELEMENTS

In addition to the standard sections of each module, there are a few other elements of treatment that may be present in each session. These elements are not included in the modules because their applications will vary widely depending on, for example, whether caregivers are included in the session and whether homework was assigned the previous week. The additional session elements are (1) weekly/daily monitoring, (2) homework review/homework assignment, and (3) setting the agenda. Each is discussed below.

Weekly/Daily Monitoring

Data from the initial assessment session(s) guide formulation of the case and inform the treatment plan. Once the plan is in motion, data are needed to tell the therapist how well the interventions are working. Regular monitoring is essential to high-quality treatment and assessment, and is described in Chapter 3.

Homework Review/Homework Assignment

There are 168 hours in each week, and usually only 1 is spent with a therapist. Thus, to help generalize what is discussed and practiced in a therapy meeting, homework is often a useful tool. Although this book does not include specific homework assignments, as those generally should be individualized to the client, a few examples are found in the different modules. A good rule of thumb for homework is to ask clients to practice using a skill outside of session. For example, for the first module (Emotion Awareness), a good homework assignment might be to play Emotion Detective at home one night with parents.

If a therapist assigns homework, reviewing it each week is critical. Doing so emphasizes a therapist's trustworthiness and consistency and also allows her the opportunity to praise the client for compliance, even if only partial compliance. Clients may find it disheartening to have invested time on a homework assignment only to have a therapist forget to ask about it.

Of course, many clients fail to complete homework assignments. Troubleshooting homework compliance could fill an entire volume, and many studies have been conducted on the subject (Houlding, Schmidt, & Walker, 2010; Hughes & Kendall, 2007). The next section details a functional analysis of homework compliance.

Functional Analysis of Homework Compliance

Step 1. Identify the Problem: Therapy Homework Compliance

Step 2. Identify Proximal Drivers

Antecedents. There are several candidates for drivers on the antecedent side. First, consider one's performance as a therapist. How well was the assignment delivered? How clear was it? Often, practicing what the homework assignment will look like can have a large impact on obtaining compliance. Below is an example of the therapist assigning homework to Brittney (the 14-year-old introduced in the previous chapter who struggles with depression and social isolation); the assignment was to involve practicing relaxation and recording before-and-after ratings.

THERAPIST: Okay, we're almost done for today. Time for the homework assignment. What do you think I'm going to ask you to do for next time?

BRITTNEY: The deep breathing and stuff we've been doing?

THERAPIST: Right! Good guess. Here's what I want you to try. First, pick one time this week when you can practice listening to the relaxation CD I made for you. You'll need a time when you have about 10 to 15 minutes and few distractions.

BRITTNEY: Maybe on Saturday would be good?

THERAPIST: Super. What time would work best, do you think?

BRITTNEY: Maybe right before I go to bed?

THERAPIST: That is a great time to practice relaxation. What time is bedtime?

BRITTNEY: 10:30 on the weekends.

THERAPIST: And will you be able to use your CD player?

BRITTNEY: Yeah.

THERAPIST: Okay, great! So, Saturday at 10 P.M., you pop in the CD. But before you press play, take a quick stress rating. Remember the stress rating?

BRITTNEY: Yeah. The 0-to-10 thing?

THERAPIST: Yep! And 10 means . . . ?

BRITTNEY: Major stress!

THERAPIST: Yep! You'll write down your rating, then press play. You'll listen to the relaxation CD. And then what?

BRITTNEY: Relax?

THERAPIST: Yes! And after the CD is over . . . ?

BRITTNEY: Write down another rating.

THERAPIST: Bingo! You would write it right here [*shows place on sheet to write the rating*]. And that's it. Then be sure to bring back the rating sheet next week so we can talk about how it went.

In some instances, a therapist might even role-play the assignment during the session—taking the prerating, simulating a relaxation period, and taking the postrating. This can be particularly helpful when the therapist anticipates low compliance or when the therapist suspects the client does not understand the assignment.

Another possible antecedent driver is the client lacking time and/or a place to complete a particular assignment. Imagine if Brittney lived in a small apartment or house and shared her bedroom with one or more siblings. Finding a private place and quiet time to practice relaxation could be a challenge. In such cases, active scouting for possible places and times to do homework may be needed, and the therapist may need to tailor certain assignments to fit the practical limitations of the child's situation. Furthermore, the therapist may need to engage the parents in the effort, as they are sometimes in a position to facilitate homework.

Another antecedent-side driver is a cognitive one. Some clients may believe that the assignment is not helpful to them—"stupid," "a waste of time," and "embarrassing"—are possible client perceptions. Most therapists who have assigned homework have heard these and worse. The interventions for such a driver are manifold. First, the therapist should ensure that the homework assignments are well designed and relevant to the child's life. Sometimes, discussing how and why the assignment is relevant convinces the client to give it a try—or the discussion could lead to the client sharing some objections that help the therapist better tailor the assignment. Second, consider alternative ways of doing the homework. If writing the assignment in a notebook or on a sheet of paper is too embarrassing for the client, then what about having her leave a voice-mail message, or send a text or e-mail? Flexibility can be helpful and is encouraged, so long as the homework provides the client an opportunity for out-of-session practice and generalization of the skills learned in treatment.

Consequences

Turning to the consequence side of the driver hunt, sometimes homework does not have enough immediate reinforcement. The therapist should plan to "shape" homework compliance rather than assume it will come of its own accord. If Brittney remembers to listen to the relaxation CD but does not record ratings, the therapist should praise the effort and move toward incorporating ratings in the next assignment. But even with rewards coming from the therapist, it is important to remember that homework assigned in treatment may not be particularly rewarding. Because therapy homework often involves challenges like talking to a new group of kids or trying a new activity, the homework itself may not lead to positive reinforcement (at least not initially). It is wise to collaborate with caregivers to identify how to reinforce clients for their homework completion. Sticker charts or point systems are effective ways to increase the probability of homework compliance.

Step 3. Gather Contextual/Situational Information

The therapist can consider whether involving others, like caregivers, is a help or hindrance. In addition, location may be relevant. For example, a client who spends some days with one parent and other days with the other parent may have very different homework compliance results depending on which house he was at before the session. One other consideration might be characteristics of the homework itself. Does assignment require the client to write something down—and what effect does that have? Some assignments might require the client to complete a task out of the home; such assignments pose logistical barriers. As may be clear from this description, the contextual factors are often ones a therapist can assess by preparing for the assignment, as was exemplified in the earlier case example. Note that the therapist determined a CD player would be present and accessible to understand how Brittney's context operated (e.g., noting the bedtime).

Step 4. Identify Distal Drivers

These could include past negative experiences with homework and schoolwork (e.g., history of not completing homework) and past negative experiences related to specific aspects of the assignment itself (e.g., assigning a client to visit a store and buy something only to learn the client once witnessed a robbery at that store), as well as any other historical factors that would contribute to the client resisting (or fearing) assignments. As described in Chapter 4, distal factors are difficult to address directly. Instead, the therapist can work with current perceptions and thoughts related to the past event. For clients whose perceptions of homework have become so negative based on what they perceive as past academic problems, therapists may choose to call the assignments by a name other than homework in order to avoid the negative connotations.

Setting the Agenda

For some therapists, setting an agenda—even *having* an agenda—may seem unfamiliar. For the modular approach described in this book, and in many evidence-based treatments, setting an agenda for each session is an integral part of structuring treatment to ensure that elements essential to treatment are provided and clients have the opportunity to contribute to the agenda overtly. The example below provides one way a therapist can set the agenda. It is worth noting that agenda setting will differ depending on who is participating in a particular session and how pressing the particular goals are. However, in general, the opening of the session involves collaborative effort to establish goals for the meeting.

THERAPIST: Sounds like the homework went pretty well. Great job remembering to take the rating after you listened to the CD. Today I thought we could talk about another skill that can sometimes be helpful when things get tough. It's called problem solving. I thought we would spend some time talking about that and practicing it. And I want to save some time at the end to hear more about that movie you were talking about when we walked in. What else would you like to put on our agenda?

BRITTNEY: I don't know. Well, maybe we can talk about my mom going on the trip and leaving me and Sal [brother] with Grandma.

THERAPIST: Let's add that to our agenda. Actually, I think we can start by talking about that now. I think it might help us think about the problem solving idea I mentioned.

In this example, the therapist adds the client's contribution to the agenda and then starts with the addition, with the aim of applying problem solving to the topic. Obviously, such an easy fit with the session's main topic is not always possible, but a review of the agenda that involves the child's input is an important part of each module.

To conclude this chapter, I provide an example of using functional analysis and modularity to plan treatment for clients.

TREATMENT PLANNING VIA FUNCTIONAL ANALYSIS

The four steps outlined in the previous section lead to a tentative conceptualization of the client's problems. A treatment plan can be built on that conceptualization through the following series of steps:

1. Prioritize the drivers.
2. Identify interventions to address the drivers.
3. Monitor progress to test the FA.
4. Repeat when necessary.

Step 1. Prioritize the Drivers

Not all drivers are created equal—some appear to exert more influence than others on a particular behavior. The goal here is to rank drivers based on their relative potency in driving the problem behaviors. The two examples below illustrate how this ranking takes place.

The first case involves 12-year-old Craig, who is missing a lot of school. Several proximal drivers are identified. The primary driver appears to be worry about his father, who has a serious illness. Craig prefers to be home so that he can be nearby to help his father, whom he perceives as needing assistance and support. The second driver is related to his parents' inconsistent responses to his school absences. At first they emphasized the importance of attending school. Then the boy's anxiety symptoms on the drive to school began to frighten his mother so much that she started regularly bringing Craig back home again, thinking he could not "handle things." Thus the second driver is succinctly: mother reinforces Craig's avoidance. Note here that the mother herself may be conceptualized as an establishing operation rather than a driver, as the boy's resistance to attending school may (and does, as it turns out) differ depending on who drives him to school. The third driver is the school's offer of a home-schooling alternative for the boy (i.e., school reinforces avoidance). The final driver is the challenging nature of the boy's schoolwork, which makes the experience of school more stressful and less pleasant than it would be if the work were less challenging. Briefly, schoolwork is a punisher.

With this conceptualization, the therapist might prioritize the child's worry and the mother's reinforcement of the avoidance and intervene by addressing the worry through cognitive work with the client and the family and working with the parents to establish a plan for reinforcing school attendance and actively ignoring client upset about attending school. The rationale for this prioritization is that both drivers appear potent and both are addressable by the therapist. Working with the school to address the third driver (school reinforces avoidance) is also possible, although not all schools are willing to collaborate. The fourth driver (schoolwork is a punisher) could be addressed by hiring an after-school tutor; however, in this case it was apparent that even if the difficulty of schoolwork were decreased, the client's worry would remain.

A second case example is that of 7-year-old Trina, with extreme levels of misbehavior including disobedience, arguing, frequent temper tantrums, and destructiveness. Several proximal drivers were identified as primary at the outset:

1. Limited parental attention for positive behavior (i.e., no one paid her much attention when she was being "good").
2. Reinforcement in the form of attention (albeit usually yelling) for "bad" behaviors (i.e., the primary time she received attention was when she had misbehaved).
3. Unclear parental instructions (i.e., when her parents did ask her to do something, their instruction was unclear ["Be a good girl"] or did not sound like a direction ["Do you want to clean your room?"]).
4. When she did behave badly, threats of punishment were rarely carried out.

Distal drivers for the case included:

1. Client temperament
2. Client ADHD
3. Parent history of poor parenting models

For this case, prioritizing the proximal drivers poses a challenge because the drivers are interrelated. However, all four drivers suggest a similar treatment direction: modification of parental behavior.

Step 2. Identify Interventions

Once the drivers are prioritized, the next step is to generate hypotheses about which interventions would influence the drivers, thereby changing (and improving) the problem behaviors. It is important to note the choice of words here: *generate hypotheses*. These ideas will be guesses, and remaining aware that they are guesses is important so that the therapist can remain open to the possibility of having guessed incorrectly or having formulated an incomplete conceptualization. Overconfidence in a treatment plan based on faulty hypotheses can lead to persistence with a bad plan, which is likely to produce a poor outcome for the client.

As an example consider Trina, the 7-year-old described earlier who had problems with disobedience. As noted, the drivers were largely related to parental behaviors. Thus interventions to address those were most likely going to involve working toward changes in parental behavior. There were relevant antecedent-related behaviors (i.e., helping the parents learn to issue more effective directions) as well as consequence-related behaviors (i.e., helping the parents to reward positive behaviors, ignore minor inappropriate ones, and effectively punish serious negative behaviors). A treatment plan for Trina would involve interventions designed to address both sets of behaviors, but a question arises: What order is the best order in which to deliver the interventions?

When multiple drivers are arguably primary and the ordering of treatment strategies is unclear, there are four possibilities to consider. First, one could examine the evidence-based treatments for the problem area(s) and ask, "What is the order of strategies in those treatment manuals?" If there is a typical sequence, there may be merit in following that order. For Trina, the therapist could have examined the disruptive behavior-disorder treatment literature. Here, the therapist would have found that many evidence-based treatment programs start with positive reinforcement strategies, like teaching parents to praise their children and to reward them for positive behaviors.

A second possibility would be to start "positive," and aim for strategies that either emphasize positive reinforcement or build on client strengths. For Trina, the emphasis would again be to teach the parents about praise and rewards, consistent with the way EBTs are organized.

Third, the therapist could start with an intervention that would have a big impact on the client's behavior. For example, in treatment for children with depression, problem solving and activity selection are often good first interventions because they both have the potential to make immediate and instrumental impact.

Finally, the therapist could ask the family members for input as to which driver is most pertinent. Doing so has the added benefit of helping keep the treatment relevant to the family's perceptions about what the problem situation really is. This strategy does run the risk of allowing families to identify a relatively less pertinent problem, either because the family doesn't know what problem is most pertinent or because the family doesn't want the therapist to know.

Obviously, consideration of all four possibilities for ranking drivers may be the optimal strategy.

Step 3. Monitor Progress

The next step is to implement the treatment plan and monitor client progress by collecting data on how the child is doing. Chapter 3 provides a discussion of assessment. Suffice it to say here that the data collected as part of treatment help guide the constantly evolving conceptualization of the case. If the data show that the problem is improving, then the conceptualization may have been accurate and the plan can be continued. If the problem does not improve, or if it worsens, then it is time to troubleshoot the conceptualization and consider revising the plan.

Step 4. Repeat When Necessary

Treatment planning based on an FA conceptualization is an iterative process by design. Drivers are listed and prioritized, interventions are identified and implemented to address the drivers, and progress is monitored. The process is more circular than linear, though. Some drivers are only identified after several weeks of treatment, leading to changes in the interventions used. Thus the last step is to reconsider all previous steps in light of new data. In the end, the idea is to continue with treatment until gains are complete.

A related point concerns emergent data. The therapist must usually create the initial conceptualization early in treatment. At our training clinic at VCU, for example, the goal is to have a treatment plan by the end of the fourth meeting, and ideally even sooner. Many clinical settings allow even less time for an initial assessment. Often, though, the early conceptualization has flaws and is marred by gaps in information. The beauty of functional analysis is that as data emerge later, they can be integrated into the conceptualization. Some new data may be consistent with the conceptualization and thus enhance confidence in the plan. Other new data may contradict the conceptualization, or, as is often the case, reveal areas not adequately considered. Being able to let go of aspects of the initial conceptualization when new data emerge is a critical skill to cultivate. The upshot is that FA is an assessment technology capable of adapting in real time if the therapist is flexible, which makes functional assessment an excellent tool for the dynamic nature of clinical work.

PUTTING IT ALL TOGETHER: CHAD AND BRITTNEY

Recall the cases of Chad and Brittney, introduced in Chapter 4. For each case, a functional analysis was generated. FA represents one method for ordering modules when applying modularity to treatment planning, and it is the method that will be used in this book. There are alternative methods, of course, including what has been referred to as a "default formulation" approach (cf. Chorpita, 2007) wherein modules are ordered in a default manner, often guided by treatment programs with an evidence base. These default formulations can be reordered in response to case realities using a set of prescribed flowcharts. Because this is a book about emotion-relevant interventions, the following two examples focus on those interventions, largely excluding discussion of other potential interventions.

Case 1: Chad

Chad is the 9-year-old boy presenting for treatment with behavioral issues at home and at school.

Step 1. Prioritize the Drivers

First, recall the hypothesized drivers identified in Chapter 4: (1) triggered when his desires are blocked (i.e., frustration tolerance); (2) thoughts or beliefs about the effectiveness of force or arguing; (3) thoughts about his not being good at tough situations; (4) triggered when he perceives he is threatened by a peer; (5) experiences difficulties when he experiences intense emotion; (6) more upset when not having discussed tough experiences from the day; (7) parental reinforcement of his misbehavior; (8) lack of parental punishment of misbehavior; (9) peer reinforcement of misbehavior; and (10) lack of parental teaching on emotion. There are numerous ways to prioritize the drivers for a case, as described earlier. For the purposes of the book, assume that an emphasis on emotional development was deemed to have primacy. Thus the drivers like low frustration tolerance, difficulty managing intense emotions, and upset when he has not discussed challenges from his day, along with the supposition that there has been limited parental teaching regarding emotion, are all prioritized.

Step 2. Identify Interventions to Address the Drivers

Given the prioritized drivers, emotion awareness, emotion understanding, and emotion regulation skills are all apparently lacking. This hypothesis has an important alternate to consider: reticence could also explain Chad's lack of emotion talk. If so, he may know how he feels and simply be unwilling to share. However, his behavior implies that either he does not know his feelings, or he knows his feelings but does not or cannot translate that knowledge into coping. Thus strong emotion regulation skills are also lacking. Accordingly, Chad may benefit from several of the modules in this book, including Module 1. Emotion Awareness Skills, Module 2. Emotion Understanding Skills, Module 6. Emotion Regulation Skills III: Expression Skills, and Module 8. Emotion Regulation Skills V: Emotion-Specific Cognitive Skills. Furthermore, given the apparent lack of parental teaching, involvement of the mother (and father, if possible) would be strongly recommended.

Selection of interventions to address the other drivers is beyond the scope of this book.

Step 3. Monitor Progress to Test the Functional Analysis

Recall that an FA is a hypothesis (or set of hypotheses) about why a client is experiencing the difficulties he is. In Chad's case, if the driver-related hypotheses are accurate, then interventions that reduce the influence of the drivers should also reduce the problematic behaviors. To test that hypothesis, Chad's therapist would need to track Chad's behaviors: arguments, tantrums, bullying behaviors, and expression of his emotions. To the extent that these indicators showed improvement, the therapist could consider the functional analysis as accurate. However, if the problem behaviors persist or worsen, then a revision of the functional analysis is needed.

Chad's entire FA, including interventions, is summarized in Figure 5.1.

Case 2: Brittney

Brittney is the 14-year-old living with her mother and younger brother. She spends a lot of time alone in her room ruminating about social interactions with peers, and she is experiencing symptoms of depression, anxiety, and social phobia.

Step 1. Prioritize the Drivers

First, recall the hypothesized drivers identified in Chapter 4: (1) triggered by others' distress, (2) expectation that others will view her negatively, (3) current adverse peer events, (4) "rewarded" by peers for having problems, (5) negative thoughts are "rewarded," and (6) lack of exposure to "contrary" evidence about her thoughts. Furthermore, as reflected in Figure 5.2, Brittney has been described as a sensitive young girl who is easily upset and hard to soothe. Temperamentally, then, Brittney is a highly emotional and sensitive teenager. Again, for the purposes of the book, an emphasis on emotional development was deemed to have primacy. Thus the prioritized primary drivers are (1) Brittney is upset by others' distress, (2) she is hypothesized to have a temperamentally high level of emotion to understand and manage, and (3) she has a lot of self-defeating thoughts that lead to her own distress.

Problems	1. Argues and throws tantrums to get his way (at home)	2. Bullies and intimidates to get his way (at school)	3. Does not understand or will not express his internal emotional state
Proximal drivers (antecedents)	Desires blocked Thoughts or beliefs (e.g., about the effectiveness of force or arguing, about his not being good at tough situations)	Desires blocked Thoughts or beliefs (e.g., about the effectiveness of force or arguing, about his not being good at tough situations) Threatened by a peer	Experiences intense emotion Not having discussed tough experiences from the day
Proximal drivers (consequences)	Parental reinforcement of misbehavior Lack of parental punishment of misbehavior	Peer reinforcement of misbehavior Lack of parental punishment of misbehavior	Lack of parental teaching on emotion
Contextual/ situational factors	When father is not present Diagnosis of ADHD	When around a large number of peers Diagnosis of ADHD	Diagnosis of ADHD
Distal drivers			Poor family emotion socialization
Interventions	**Module 6. Emotion Regulation Skills III: Expression Skills**	**Module 6. Emotion Regulation Skills III: Expression Skills**	**Module 1. Emotion Awareness Skills** **Module 2. Emotion Understanding Skills** **Module 8. Emotion Regulation Skills V: Emotion-Specific Cognitive Skills (with a focus on anger for Chad)**

FIGURE 5.1. Chad's functional analysis with treatment plan.

Step 2. Identify Interventions to Address the Drivers

Given the prioritized drivers, emotion awareness, empathy, and emotion regulation skills are all identified as key foci for treatment. Accordingly, as reflected in Figure 5.2, the modules focusing on those topics were chosen to guide treatment. The three most applicable emotion regulation modules are Module 4. Emotion Regulation Skills I: Prevention Skills, which focuses on reducing susceptibility to emotional experiences; Module 7. Emotion Regulation Skills IV: Basic Cognitive Skills, designed to help Brittney manage her thoughts about situations that tend to escalate her emotional distress; and Module 8. Emotion Regulation Skills V: Emotion-Specific Cognitive Skills, designed to help Brittney manage thoughts related to specific emotions, such as sadness. As in Chad's case, selecting interventions to address the other drivers is beyond the scope of this book. However, it is worth noting that the emotion regulation modules also could have a positive effect on some of the other drivers.

Step 3. Monitor Progress to Test the Functional Analysis

As with Chad's case, Brittney's therapist would need to track her behaviors and note the extent to which improvement is achieved. Lack of improvement would suggest the need to revisit the FA and reconsider the treatment plan.

Brittney's entire FA, including interventions, is summarized in Figure 5.2.

CONCLUSION

Combining FA with modularity represents a potentially fruitful integration. Although this chapter focused on treatment planning involving emotion-related interventions, the combination of FA and modularity has a broader application. Indeed, as noted, a recent study by Weisz and colleagues (2012) found that the modular approach was superior to standard manualized approaches as well as usual care. This study included children with primary problems of anxiety, depression, or disruptive behavior and was conducted in community clinics in two large, diverse metropolitan areas (Boston, Massachusetts, and Honolulu, Hawaii). A preliminary test of the application of functional analysis in conjunction with modularity has just been completed (see Southam-Gerow et al., 2009, for description). Thus the approach described in this chapter represents the cutting edge of science in the area of child mental health.

Problems	1. High levels of depressed mood	2. Overfocus on negative events (rumination)	3. Social isolation
Proximal drivers (antecedents)	Others' distress Expects others to view her negatively	Adverse peer events Others' distress Expects others to view her negatively	Adverse peer events Expects others to view her negatively
Proximal drivers (consequences)	"Rewarded" by peers for problems	"Rewarded" by peers for problems Negative thoughts are "rewarded" Lack of exposure to "contrary" evidence	 Negative thoughts are "rewarded" Lack of exposure to "contrary" evidence
Contextual/ situational factors	Relative absence of adult support Temperamental vulnerability to others' distress Predisposition to depression	Relative absence of adult support Temperamental vulnerability to others' distress Predisposition to depression	Relative absence of adult support Temperamental vulnerability to others' distress Predisposition to depression
Distal drivers	 Parents' divorce	 Parents' divorce	Mother's experience in a depressed family Parents' divorce
Interventions	**Module 1. Emotion Awareness Skills** **Module 4. Emotion Regulation Skills I: Prevention Skills** **Module 8. Emotion Regulation Skills V: Emotion-Specific Cognitive Skills**	**Module 3. Empathy Skills** **Module 7. Emotion Regulation Skills IV: Basic Cognitive Skills**	 **Module 7. Emotion Regulation Skills IV: Basic Cognitive Skills**

FIGURE 5.2. Brittney's functional analysis with treatment plan.

CHAPTER 6

Final Considerations
Caregivers, Culture, and Engaging Challenging Clients

Clients (and friends) are often surprised when I fail to have specific answers to questions they have about their children. "Is it normal that my daughter doesn't invite friends over to hang out?" or "What should I do about my son? He's always making his friends mad at him." Training as a mental health professional does not (in my opinion) give access to clear answers to these or many other burning questions. Instead, our training affords a breadth of knowledge on adaptive and maladaptive development, as well as a method for trying out ideas that *could* be helpful in solving thorny dilemmas. The method asks the mental health professional to (1) consider each person involved and his or her individual characteristics, (2) consider the context in which the problem is occurring, (3) devise a plan to solve the problem, and (4) collect data to know whether that plan has worked or is working. This idea probably makes good sense to most readers, but some clients (and friends) react to the approach with frustration: "You mental health people never want to give a straight answer!"

It's true: there are rarely clear answers to the problems that clients bring in, especially when the question concerns how to help facilitate emotional development in children and adolescents. Human development and adaptation are nuanced and rarely lend themselves to simple prescriptions. This chapter explores three topics that make delivering emotion-informed interventions to children and adolescents such a fascinating challenge: (1) parent/caregiver involvement, (2) ethnic and cultural diversity, and (3) engaging challenging clients.

PARENT/CAREGIVER INVOLVEMENT

The reasons to involve caregivers in treatment are many. First, caregivers are primary sources of information about our young clients, some of whom cannot or will not provide valid data on what ails them. Relatedly, because caregivers are generally the referring individuals and nearly always the people paying for treatment, their involvement is critical because they are the customers, so to speak. In addition, caregivers are among the (if not *the*) most important and influential individuals in the life of the client, and as such can be extremely helpful in promoting change in the client's life. Finally, understanding and adjusting caregiver's *contributions* to a client's difficulties is often a key focus of intervention. Indeed, there are entire brands of treatment predicated on the notion that the family is the unit of intervention.

An argument can also be made against involving caregivers in treatment. First, data supporting its efficacy are relatively limited for some problem areas. For example, for anxiety and depression (Chorpita & Southam-Gerow, 2006; Stark et al., 2006), there are data to suggest that individually focused treatments work just as well as treatments involving caregivers. None of the studies to date have completely eliminated caregiver involvement from treatment, and many are not particularly specific about how caregivers are involved. Data suggest that *routine caregiver involvement*, such as chatting for a few minutes at the start and end of meetings with the child, appears to produce similarly positive effects when compared to more intensive and structured caregiver involvement (e.g., Chorpita & Southam-Gerow, 2006; Stark et al., 2006).

A second, albeit limited, argument against caregiver involvement is the fact that some caregivers prefer not to be involved, believing that therapy is something the child receives much in the way that he receives piano or karate lessons. In this case, involving caregivers means having to sell them on the rationale for their involvement. Ultimately, this is *not* an argument against involving caregivers so much as an acknowledgement that, in some cases, involving them is a challenge because of their own limited motivation. A therapist may be tempted to not involve a caregiver because of her avoidance of opportunities to become involved. In such cases, rather than insist on caregiver involvement to proceed, it is perhaps more prudent to pursue caregiver engagement while tracking client outcomes, to discern whether the lack of caregiver involvement is truly hindering progress.

A third argument is purely practical: there are some treatment settings that make caregiver involvement particularly challenging or impossible. For example, more and more mental health care is provided in schools during the school day, often limiting the involvement of caregivers, many of whom work during school hours.

In the end, despite these counterarguments, pursuit of caregiver involvement is a laudable and generally warranted goal. The upsides to engaging caregivers often outweigh the downsides. One may ask, "How can I justify not involving a person who is with the client most often and most intensely?" In the next section, a few examples of caregiver-related drivers that would warrant considerable caregiver involvement are described, focusing primarily on emotion-informed interventions.

Reasons to Involve Caregivers in Emotion-Focused Treatment

Caregiver Knowledge Gap

Lack of knowledge about emotion development can be an important driver for considering caregiver involvement. Mental health providers often take their knowledge for granted. Even well-educated caregivers rarely possess the specific expertise that most mental health providers have concerning mental health and child development. Sharing that knowledge can be powerful. The good news is that, for some caregivers, information alone may be adequate. Armed with information about emotional development and how to help their children develop emotion regulation skills, some caregivers may make changes to their parenting behavior that will reap significant benefits. For example, some data suggest that providing educational support groups for caregivers of children with anxiety disorders can be beneficial; one possible reason for this is that if caregivers receive information about the problem, they may be able to figure out how to solve it (e.g., Chorpita & Daleiden, 2009).

Caregiver Knowledge and Skill Gaps

A more common driver is a combination of both knowledge and skill gaps. It is important to distinguish skill gaps from more toxic parenting situations discussed below. Consider Tara, an 11-year-old with anxiety and budding depressive symptoms. Her mother was divorced, worked long hours, and had little energy to parent. Tara learned early on to stay out of trouble, but as she grew older and her social world became more complicated, she began to find it more challenging to grapple with her emotional world. Because her mother was stretched thin, Tara was loath to burden her mother with her emotions. In addition, her mother had never really learned how to talk about her own emotions and thus had limited skills for doing so with her daughter; Tara had little opportunity to practice emotion talk and was exposed to very little modeling of how one does so. A difference between Tara's mother and the caregivers discussed in the next section is that once Tara's mother understood the possible benefits of promoting Tara's emotional development, she made some efforts to change her own behavior with assistance from the therapist.

Caregiver Knowledge and Skill Gaps Plus . . .

The most problematic of the three caregiver-related drivers is the caregiver who not only has knowledge and skills gaps, but who also engages in toxic emotional interactions and/or is strongly against the notion that his/her own behaviors are related to the child's difficulties. Most readers will have several such cases that come to mind immediately. Consider this example.

Shelly was a 14-year-old who lived part-time with her mother and part-time with her father and her stepmother. She presented with anxiety symptoms, including some perfectionistic tendencies in schoolwork and social anxieties. She was also worried a lot about her mother. As it turned out, some of the worry for her mother was warranted insofar as Shelly's mother had been diagnosed with bipolar disorder and borderline personality disorder. The mother's interactions with Shelly were sometimes positive and loving; however, there were many times when the mother would engage in behaviors such as denigrating Shelly for particular emotional states (e.g., mocking her when she was feeling stressed about schoolwork), ignoring Shelly when she tried to share her emotions, and alternately raging and weeping to Shelly (i.e., demonstrating emotion dysregulation). What made these distressing events particularly challenging was that Shelly's mother had almost no insight into how her own behaviors were affecting her daughter.

Cases like these are no-brainers when it comes to answering the questions *Does the caregiver's behavior contribute to the problems?* and *Would the client benefit if the caregiver were involved in treatment?* And yet they are the toughest when it comes to identifying ways to involve the caregiver and promote change. In the next section, some strategies are described that can assist therapists in engaging caregivers.

Strategies for Engaging Caregivers

If the therapist has chosen to involve the caregiver(s), the next question is *how* to involve him/her/them. The case conceptualization will drive how (and how much) caregivers are involved. In Chapter 4, I outlined the functional analytic approach to case conceptualization, in which the goal was to identify a deep understanding of the drivers or contributors to the client's problems. With the case conceptualization in mind, there are several types of caregiver involvement to consider, arranged here in their order of intensity from lowest to highest: (1) outcome monitoring, (2) support of therapy progress, (3) parallel work, and (4) concurrent work.

Outcome Monitoring

At a minimum, outcome monitoring is an important way to involve nearly all caregivers. Asking them how the client is doing, and relying on idiographic and standardized measures, should be considered a minimum standard of care. Given the likelihood that the caregiver was the person who initiated therapy, the caregiver's sense of how things are going is essential. One may choose to continue past this level of involvement, but in some cases monitoring may be all that is necessary or possible.

Support of Therapy Progress

At the second level of intensity, the therapist can invest time and effort to ensure that caregivers understand what the client is working on in therapy meetings. This involvement needs to consider client confidentiality, of course. In many cases, the therapist will want to emphasize how the caregiver can prompt and help generalize any skills the client has been learning in therapy. Involvement with and support of therapy homework is an obvious application, but the benefits of caregivers knowing what their child is working on in therapy go beyond the increased chances of homework compliance. The better caregivers understand the focus of therapy, the more likely they will be to support that focus in the more than 160 hours per week that the client is not working with the therapist.

This level of intensity in caregiver involvement is relatively common and can be more or less formal, ranging from a few minutes in the waiting room to 10 minutes or so of face-to-face meeting time, with occasional full-length caregiver-only meetings. Most of the meetings are focused on the child. A common strategy is for the therapist and client reconnect with the caregiver(s) at the end of a child session, updating the caregiver(s) on progress and what the client will be working on during the upcoming week.

Parallel Work

Another notch up in intensity involves doing parallel work with client and caregiver. For example, the therapist could divide a meeting time into two segments, one working with the caregiver and the other working with the child. Alternatively, meetings could switch every other week: one week with just the child, and the next with just the caregiver. Whatever the arrangement, the goal is to engage both the caregiver and the client in work that is separate but designed to help the child.

Any of the modules in the book could be presented in parallel fashion. In parallel meetings, there is often a different emphasis with caregivers than with the child. For example, with the child, the therapist may discuss different ways to regulate emotion and then practice some of the ideas generated. With the parent, the therapist may emphasize education on emotion regulation and then initiate a conversation about how the caregiver can nurture the child's burgeoning efforts to regulate emotion more adaptively.

An important advantage of parallel (vs. conjoint) meetings is that a caregiver may feel more comfortable speaking freely, especially regarding his or her contributions to the child's problems. Taking time to discuss and think through these contributions can be valuable, but therapists are wise to guard against becoming the caregiver's therapist. To maintain a focus on the client (vs. the parent), the therapist may need to remind the caregiver gently about the child focus. Having a good set of referrals for caregivers is also advisable for cases where a caregiver may benefit from individual therapy.

Concurrent Work

Concurrent (or conjoint) work is not necessarily a more intense level of parent involvement. In many cases, parallel and concurrent sessions end up with the therapist spending approximately the same amount of time with a caregiver. Instead, concurrent sessions permit a different sort of meeting, one that (1) focuses most of the attention on the child and on parent–child interaction, (2) allows practice of skills learned immediately, permitting therapist feedback to both client and caregiver, and (3) provides enhanced support for the client as she attempts to learn the emotional development skills covered by the modules in this book. This enhanced support may be particularly beneficial for younger clients whose attention spans and/or retention abilities are relatively limited.

Although one might use the same module in parallel and concurrent meetings, there is an important distinction in the method of presentation. In concurrent meetings, the caregiver is generally viewed as a therapist aide and/or home coach; the therapist and caregiver collaborate to teach the client the content of the module.

When the case conceptualization suggests that caregiver-related drivers go beyond the *knowledge gap* level, a good rule of thumb is to aim for a mix of the latter three intensity levels (support of therapy progress, parallel work, and concurrent work). Some messages are best delivered in parallel meetings, whereas others lend themselves better the conjoint meetings. A few specific guidelines to note:

1. With *younger children* (about 8 years and under), a strong dose of conjoint meetings, along with some parallel meetings, is often useful. Younger children sometimes struggle in "talk" therapy, even when toys and play are used. Including the caregiver may increase the child's comfort. Furthermore, the caregiver is present to add his or her perspective to the therapist's questions.
2. With *older children* (usually 13 and up), parallel meetings are often useful, as individual meetings may increase the chances that the child will confide in the therapist. Furthermore, such a structure supports the normative striving for autonomy.
3. With *tweens* (ages 9 to 12), some combination of the first two approaches is likely to be appropriate. Because development is so variable for this age group in particular, there is no clear rule of thumb.
4. With *particularly difficult caregivers*, parallel meetings may be a good idea to provide additional support to the caregiver while reducing the chances of having meetings in which the caregiver dominates the discussion with his or her own issues and/or complaints about the child in front of the child.

The form and goals of caregiver involvement will vary depending on the needs of the child. In the end, though, given the critical importance of caregivers as emotional educators for their children, involving caregivers in emotion-informed interventions for children is nearly always a good idea.

ETHNIC AND CULTURAL DIVERSITY
AND THEIR RELATION TO EMOTION

Emotions have strong physiological bases, with roots in the central and peripheral nervous systems. However, as discussed in Chapter 2, emotions are also social constructs, and as such, there are important variants of emotional experience across cultures. Fostering emotional development requires a therapist to understand and embrace diversity. In this brief section, I discuss different ways in which culture may influence emotion—and how therapists aiming to use emotion-informed interventions might proceed in a culturally sensitive way.

Research on culture and emotion relies on early theoretical and empirical work by Geert Hofstede (e.g., Hofstede, Hofstede, & Minkov, 2010) and Harry Triandis (e.g., Triandis, 1995), and more recently on David Matsumoto's (e.g., Matsumoto & Hwang, 2012) empirical work. Although culture has been defined as composed of many dimensions relevant for emotion development, the most often studied dimension is that of collectivism versus individualism. An *individualist* culture emphasizes the needs and desires of the individual; it places high value on personal time, freedom, challenge, and such extrinsic motivators as material rewards at work. In family relations, individualist cultures value honesty/truth, talking things out, using guilt to achieve behavioral goals, and maintaining self-respect. Finally, individualist cultures emphasize self-actualization and self-realization.

Collectivist cultures emphasize the needs and desires of the collective or group, be it the family group or larger groups, such as groups defined culturally or via other means (e.g., work groups). There is a strong value placed on harmonious relations over absolute honesty. Finally, collectivist cultures emphasize harmony, consensus, and equality.

These broadly defined cultural perspectives have implications for emotional competence generally, and more specifically for aspects of emotional competence such as emotional expression and the experience of specific emotions. A discussion of these issues is beyond the scope of this chapter, and the interested reader is referred to Triandis's (1995) classic book. Instead, the following discussion focuses on the clinical implications of potential cultural differences in emotional competence.

A therapist using emotion-informed interventions should consider several cultural points before proceeding. First and perhaps foremost, he must recognize and become highly aware of the cultural frame through which he observes and judges a client's interactions and emotion-related displays. A therapist's own cultural background and experiences influence how he understands emotions, and that background can blind him to a client's actual experiences. Consulting other sources for more in-depth information about culture and its impact on emotional development is strongly recommended. In addition, it can be useful to talk with clients and their families about the families' cultures and how culture influences how the family thinks about emotions. Such conversations can help build an understanding of the clients' families' microculture(s) in a way that can be more helpful and relevant than general readings on cultural competence.

A second important point is that a therapist should not assume that open and clear expression of emotions is a goal that all families will endorse. Therapists are encouraged to engage families in a discussion about when emotion expression is acceptable and desirable, focusing on the family's understanding of how and when emotion should be expressed, and respecting differences that arise. Therapists may choose to share what they know about the importance of expressing (vs. not expressing) feelings for physical and mental health, as well as the importance of regulating emotional expression in a contextually sensitive way. At the same time, therapists should remember that research on the benefits of emotion expression is limited, particularly as it relates to culture. An important aim here is to identify how to tailor the content of an intervention for families whose cultural values may lean toward one end or the other of the spectrum of emotion regulation (i.e., cultures that emphasize and value ample emotional expression vs. those that emphasize and value more limited emotional expression).

Although emotions represent universal experiences relevant to successful adaptation around the world, there are important cultural moderators of emotion. Implementing emotion-related interventions with families and children requires a sensitive and culturally competent stance.

STRATEGIES FOR ENGAGING DIFFICULT CLIENTS

Many clients have trouble getting started talking about their feelings. Some have never been exposed to emotion talk in their homes, while others have only been exposed to select emotional topics, like happiness or anger. Still others have better exposure to emotion language but hesitate to discuss their feelings due to a range of expectations about what might happen if they do talk about their feelings. Below are profiles of several types of challenging clients. For each category, some troubleshooting strategies are offered.

The Shy/Reticent Client

First, there is the client who is reticent but not oppositional. These clients often have the inhibited temperamental style Jerome Kagan has described as the tendency to withdraw from novel or social experiences (e.g., Kagan et al., 1994). One important caveat made especially relevant in light of the previous section on culture: it is important to distinguish those clients who are temperamentally shy from those whose cultural background calls on them to appear shy, at least when interacting with authority figures.

Assuming the client really is reticent, it can be helpful for the therapist to do some talking. It is important to be clear here: understanding clients' experiences requires the therapist to do more listening than speaking. However, long pauses and open-ended questions can create tremendous anxiety for some reticent clients. In these cases, waiting for the client to be ready to talk can potentially make things worse. If the therapist does the lion's share of the talking at first, she can model what talking in therapy sounds like while normalizing some of the client's experiences. Furthermore, the therapist's talking may take some of the heat off the client, allowing him to settle into the relationship without feeling he must open up completely and immediately. As treatment proceeds, the therapist can move toward greater client participation.

Reticent clients sometimes feel more comfortable talking and participating when the situation does not follow the typical one-on-one, face-to-face therapeutic interaction model. Instead, a therapist can conduct therapy while walking, playing a game, drawing, or engaging in almost any activity. Indeed, many children, regardless of how shy, are not comfortable or equipped for the intense *talking* that therapists do with many adult clients. Sometimes the best sessions take place during a kickball game in a hallway or on a walk around the neighborhood.

The Hit-or-Miss Client

A second challenging client is one who is more easily engaged than the shy/reticent client, but mostly on issues of no apparent clinical import. Such clients use a variety of methods to demonstrate their unwillingness to talk about certain topics. Distraction is a common go-to strategy for this client. Consider Angel, a 13-year old who is chatty on most topics, especially movies and music; however, when her family comes up, she changes the topic so swiftly and easily that in the beginning the therapist didn't even notice. Another strategy of the hit-or-miss client is to clam up. But in contrast to the shy/reticent client who appears visibly anxious, the hit-or-miss client seems annoyed and perhaps even angry. There is a withholding quality for the hit-or-miss client that is absent in the shy/reticent client. It may seem like the hit-or-miss client can talk but refuses to do so, whereas the shy/reticent client fears talking or may even believe that he truly cannot talk about the subject at hand.

So what to do with a hit-or-miss client? One strategy is called the *back-pocket kid*, also known as the "I have a friend who . . . " technique. Here, the therapist engages in a conversation or exercise pertinent to the client's issues without requiring the client to acknowledge that the conversation is applicable to her life. For example, with 13-year-old Angel described above, the therapist could describe a 14-year-old kid he knows named Julia who has trouble talking with her mother. He could then ask Angel how she thinks Julia could get along better with her parents. The back-pocket kid is often easier for the client to talk about than her own life.

Another way to proceed with the hit-or-miss client is through modalities alternative to talking. For example, some clients will do a lot of good work if given the opportunity to write. Others feel comfortable with various technologies such as e-mails, text messaging, or even video blogging. Still others will feel more expressive when engaged with an artistic medium like paints or crayons. The idea is to offer a variety of ways for the client to communicate and learn with you. Of course, some of these methods pose confidentiality and boundary issues that should be carefully considered. For example, if a therapist chooses to exchange e-mails with a client, steps should be taken to safeguard confidentiality (e.g., password-protected files, not using identifying information in the messages).

The Hostile Client

Hostile clients are familiar to most therapists. These are the clients who absolutely refuse to engage. It's as if the client comes into the meetings with his middle fingers in the up-and-locked position. There are a variety of reasons that a client becomes a hostile client, and understanding the reasons goes a long way toward experimenting with ideas to help the client. A good functional assessment (see Chapter 4) can help a therapist identify the optimal strategy for working with and around a client's resistance. For example, some hostile clients are upset to be the ones in treatment because they view their caregivers or others in their family as the ones with the problems. Other hostile clients have had bad experiences with therapists in the past and have adopted a no-trust policy. Still other hostile clients have a general distrust of adults or authority figures or people of your particular ethnic/cultural group or the ethnic/cultural group represented by your agency.

Once a therapist has an understanding of the reason(s) that the client is in full hostile mode, she can devise some strategies to foster a working relationship, assuming that doing so makes sense. For example, if the client has a strong preference for a therapist of a particular gender or ethnic group, one potentially effective way to acknowledge that concern would be with a referral.

Motivational enhancement is a potentially useful approach with a hostile client. This involves the client-centered strategies of empathy and mirroring, coupled with a more directive strategy aimed at identifying domains for possible change in the client's life (e.g., Miller & Rollnick, 2013). Through empathic and active listening, the therapist identifies discrepancies between the way things are and the way the client wants things to be. Therein lies the opportunity to help facilitate changes.

Orthogonal interaction techniques also may counteract the child's lack of engagement (e.g., Efran, Lukens, & Lukens, 1990). Engaging in orthogonal interactions means interacting with a client in unexpected ways such that the client has trouble responding in his characteristic way. For example, a therapist may decide to sit and work quietly at her desk after having tried and failed for several minutes to engage the hostile client in the session. Rather than engage in the pursuit–withdrawal cycle, the therapist also disengages, demonstrating to the client that she will not work if the client does not work. Some clients in this situation will ask what the therapist is doing, sometimes in a complaining way, as if to say, "Hey—we are paying for this. Why aren't you talking?" When used carefully, such approaches can help create openings to talk about the client's resistance to therapy. Therapists should be cautioned, though, that such strategies are difficult to implement well. The interested reader is referred to the work of Milton Erickson (see Haley, 1993), Jay Haley (1991), and Jay Efran (e.g., Efran et al., 1990) as exemplars of this approach.

A final idea for working with the hostile client is to work around her. Many readers are familiar with family therapy approaches that posit therapy meetings must take place with all family members in order to be effective. Some approaches assume that work with a single member of the family *reverberates* throughout the entire family. Along those lines, then, sometimes working with *others* in the family can be a way to make some positive changes in a client's life.

Working with highly resistant and openly hostile clients represents one of the biggest challenges therapists face. These brief paragraphs could not possibly depict all of the optimal methods for maximizing the effects of treatment. Readers are encouraged to consult other books and articles on engaging difficult clients and consider these ideas as just that: a few ideas to consider until better ones can be identified. Furthermore, readers are also encouraged to seek out consultation when truly "stuck" with a challenging client.

CONCLUSION

This chapter does only limited justice to three particularly important topics in clinical work with children and adolescents. Entire volumes could be (and are) written on each topic individually. And although working with caregivers, considering diversity, and engaging clients are all important for any form of therapy, they are particularly salient for emotion-informed interventions. First, as described in Chapter 2, emotions have social relevance as a child's emotional competence develops in the social world. As such, understanding caregiver influences and involving them in treatment can be critical when helping a client develop her emotional skills. And as noted in Chapter 2, emotions are partly biological, partly social, and partly cultural. Thus therapists are encouraged to consider how people of different cultural groups may experience emotions. Finally, engaging clients in talking and learning about emotions can be one of the most challenging aspects of a therapist's work. Although mental health practitioners are often comfortable talking about feelings, the penchant for doing so is less common in the general public. For all three topics, therapists are encouraged to use creativity and flexibility to find the combination of ideas that will help each client develop her emotional life as well as possible.

PART II

TREATMENT MODULES

MODULE 1

Emotion Awareness Skills

$\mathbf{E}$ach of the following chapters is organized in a modular fashion such that a therapist can use any one of the eight modules by itself during treatment. However, the eight modules are arranged in a logical, developmental, and therefore default order such that one could proceed sequentially through the modules. Hence, because this is the first module, it represents one of the earliest developmental acquisitions leading to emotional competence: emotional awareness.

The organization of all of the modules follows a format based on the one used by Chorpita (2007) in his modular approach and as described in Chapter 5 of this book.

WHEN TO USE THIS MODULE

This module is designed for use when a major contributor to a client's difficulties is a lack of skills in recognizing *his or her own* or *others'* emotions. A therapist could use data from a number of sources to arrive at this conclusion. Lack of emotional awareness skills may be inferred from how the client presents in session, although such data may be misleading. As the savvy therapist knows from training and experience, there are many reasons a client might offer little in terms of emotionally relevant conversation in a session. Thus careful attention to assessment will serve the clinician well in selection of the most appropriate and effective interventions.

One example of a client for whom this module might be selected is the soft-spoken 9-year-old, Chad, described in Chapter 4, who was referred for behavior problems at home and at school (e.g., teasing other children, defiance with mother, tantrums). Chad's functional analysis revealed two emotion-related drivers related to the topic of this module: Chad's lack of emotional vocabulary and the mismatch between Chad's apparent affect and his expressed affect. Accordingly, the Emotion Awareness Skills module would be an appropriate intervention to consider.

OBJECTIVES

Objectives for the module are to teach and practice the skills involved in being aware of our own feelings as well as the feelings of others. The three steps outlined in this module are:

1. Identifying emotions
2. Rating emotion intensity
3. Expressing emotions

The skills here are developmentally basic; as such, the module does not involve the more complex levels of emotion knowledge that are covered in the Emotion Understanding Skills or Empathy Skills modules, for example. Here the focus is on fundamental emotion knowledge: (1) that there is a range of feelings, (2) that feelings come in a range of intensities, and (3) that there is a range of ways to express those feelings.

As with all of the modules in the book, the primary recommended method for evaluating progress toward the objective is *through observation of the applied skill in the life of the client*. That is, the therapist should see how well the client "walks the walk" of emotion awareness. To do this, the therapist's own observations are used in combination with the reports from significant others in the client's life, like parents or teachers or the client him/herself.

PROCEDURES
Step 1. Identifying Emotions

Overview

The first step in the module is to teach and practice identifying emotions, in the client herself and in others. The skill is a basic one and a building block for so many of the other skills covered in this book, and yet, sadly, it is a skill many clients do not have.

Teach

Why Identifying Emotions Is Important

The rationale for learning to identify emotions or feelings is straightforward. First, emotions are an important part of getting along with others. Knowing how others feel makes us a better friend, and knowing how we feel helps us to navigate tricky times in our various relationships. Second, being able to identify one's own (and others') feelings is the first step toward being able to rate how "strong" those feelings are. Third, knowing how one feels helps one to make good choices when one experiences emotions in strong ways. Becoming proficient at identifying one's own feelings facilitates a proactive approach to one's emotional life. The more quickly a person recognizes his feelings, particularly ones that may hinder functioning, the more quickly he can cope with those feelings. Fourth, even when life turns "rotten" (as it always does from time to time), knowing how to identify our feelings can help in a few ways. For example, feelings are guides to what is important to people. So if Emmy is sad that Stan is moving away, that means Emmy cares for Stan, a fact that is good for Emmy to know, even though it makes her sad. In addition, knowing how one is feeling in tough times can help one reach out to others and express oneself, something discussed later.

Survey the Various Feelings We Experience

This teaching point has five separate subpoints: (1) there are a lot of different feelings; (2) each feeling can cause physical changes in the body, and those changes can be different across time for the same emotion and the same for different emotions; (3) some of the signs for emotions are visible, while others require one to know something "internal" (i.e., a person's attitudes or experiences) about oneself (or someone else) or to guess; (4) hiding feelings does not mean one is not feeling them; and (5) it is important to practice identifying one's own and other people's emotions.

The **Feelings, Feelings, Everywhere!** worksheet (**Handout 1**) at the end of this module is one tool, particularly useful for younger clients, to elicit a list of a variety of different emotions. The client could complete the worksheet in session individually or with the therapist's guidance, or the therapist could assign the worksheet as homework. Another worksheet, **Feelings and Our Bodies (Handout 2)**, asks clients to match up bodily sensations with their probably underlying emotions.

Practice: Activities and Games

The following set of activities and games represents a few possible ways to teach and practice the skill of identifying emotions. Though described here to help practice the "identification" skill, the games could be adapted to address the second and third steps as well.

Emotion Dictionary

This activity is ubiquitous in treatment programs and thus many therapists will be familiar with it.

Preparation. In advance of session, a therapist planning to engage in this activity will need to assemble materials for building the dictionary. Simple art supplies often suffice, although if the client will respond well to a technological version of the game, such as using photos from a digital camera, the therapist will need to have electronic supplies to upload photos to a computer.

Gameplay. The client and therapist (caregivers can also be involved) work together to create a list of emotion words. Ideally, the client does the bulk of the work; however, some clients may struggle or be reticent when listing emotions. In those cases, therapists are encouraged to contribute to the list. However, it is generally wise to pause between suggestions to see if the therapist-generated idea has inspired the client.

With the word list generated, therapist and client work on a "definition" for each word. Such a definition can take many shapes. For instance, the client can generate traditional written definitions of each word, using a dictionary if necessary. Or, instead of written definitions, the therapist and client can search for pictures in magazines that match each word. Children who enjoy drawing may choose to illustrate each word with a drawing or a scene. As noted earlier, digital photos or videos can also be taken and used.

No matter how the words are defined, the work is assembled into some collection (e.g., scrapbook, video file on computer). Once compiled, the dictionary can be revisited in later sessions for review or to add new emotions.

Feelings Detectives/Emotion Charades

This is a variation of the popular parlor game that involves acting out emotions and focuses on helping the client identify clues about another's emotional state.

Preparation. The therapist will benefit from having some index cards handy on which to write feeling words. Otherwise, this game requires very little preparation.

Gameplay. The game involves the client and therapist generating a list of emotion words, as with the emotion dictionary exercise. Each word is written on an index card. The cards are then shuffled and each person takes turns drawing a card and acting out the emotion written on the card. The involvement of caregivers can be a positive experience, permitting the therapist to assess the caregiver's own emotional awareness. As in charades, the player(s) not acting out the emotion are tasked with guessing the emotion being portrayed.

The detective aspect of the game comes in when the therapist and client identify which clues led to their guesses. The actor is encouraged to share other clues not identified by the player.

A more advanced variation of the game involves having each participant act out or describe a scene that could lead to particular feelings. Rather than relying on facial and bodily expressions, the participants must consider the goals and preferences of an individual in a situation. When playing this way, each situation can actually be "riffed" to lead to multiple feelings, depending on the variation of different factors. As an example, take a scene where a friend comes over and invites the character to ride bikes. In response to the invitation, many children will assume that the invited child will feel happy or excited. However, if one knew that the child was in a bike accident a few days earlier, how might the feelings be different? What if one knew that the child did not know how to ride a bike? Using the more advanced variation is good for older children, helps teach perspective-taking skills, and emphasizes the point that feelings are not only what one might see reflected in a person's face or body.

The following example depicts this game with 14-year-old Tyiesha.

THERAPIST: Let's play another game. In this game, I'll act out a scene and you'll try to use your feelings detective skills we just talked about to figure out how I am feeling. Here we go . . . I am in school and the teacher has just announced a big test. *(Groans and clutches stomach, wipes her hands on her pants, and furrows her brow.)*

TYIESHA: You are feeling worried? It looks like your face is squinched up.

THERAPIST: Good; what else do you notice? *(Resumes the scene.)*

TYIESHA: You are touching your stomach. Maybe you have a funny feeling there? You look stressed in your face. Oh, and your hands—you're wiping them. Maybe they're sweaty?

THERAPIST: Great—you get the idea. I was feeling worried. And you noticed the clues in my face, in the way I was rubbing my hands, and how I seemed to have a stomachache. Now let's try a different one. This time, you play the person having the feeling. Let's say you're at school. I'm your friend and you're telling me about something upsetting that happened to you. We'll play that scene out a little bit and then each do some detective work to figure out how each of us has been feeling. Ready?

TYIESHA: Wait, I'm going to be complaining about something bad that happened—like what?

THERAPIST: What do you think would be good?

TYIESHA: Maybe my other friend was pretty mean to me on the bus?

THERAPIST: Ouch! That would be upsetting—Let's try it!

TYIESHA: Okay.

[After acting out the scene . . .]

THERAPIST: Okay, let me see if I can guess what you were feeling. You seemed sad, I think, cause you were sniffling like you might cry and your eyes were squinting. And what you were saying made me think you were sad. I must have missed something? What else were you doing?

> Tyiesha: You did good. I was also feeling that bad feeling in my stomach, like I just got punched, but maybe you couldn't tell. I talked quieter too.
>
> Therapist: You did talk quieter—that's right. And you are right on that I couldn't tell your stomach felt upset. Good work, Tyiesha!

The focus of the activity does not need to be solely on physiological emotional reactions. For example, in addition to noting that her face gets hot and her hands may clench when she feels angry, the therapist can also note that anger often comes in response to feeling tricked, misunderstood, or even nervous. The key here is to work with the client to identify ways of knowing when he is feeling a particular way, as well as to recognize others' feelings, with the rationale that doing so helps the client to cope better with those feelings.

For this activity, using scenes that are not so close to the client's own experience may be helpful, so long as they offer the opportunity to teach emotion skills. Furthermore, the therapist can start the game by talking about the feelings of others rather than the client's own feelings. However, as the client becomes more comfortable with the game, the therapist should move into more personal situations. A final case example, involving Tyiesha again, illustrates how one might accomplish that goal.

> Therapist: Okay, next let's try something that happened to you recently. What feeling should we start with?
>
> Tyiesha: Oh, I don't know. Happy?
>
> Therapist: Great idea. Okay, think of a time you were happy lately and then we can do the scene and play feelings detectives.
>
> Tyiesha: Okay—well, the other day, my mom made my favorite dinner—spaghetti with meatballs. I felt happy.
>
> Tyiesha: Okay, good one. I will be your mom and I am serving up dinner. Let's see if I can tell that you are happy.
>
> *[After role play . . .]*
>
> Therapist: Okay, let's see if I can detect the clues that would tell us you were happy. First, I noticed that you smiled. It wasn't a huge smile, but sometimes teenagers don't smile widely. *(Tyiesha laughs.)* Also, you said that you liked the meal.
>
> Tyiesha: Yeah. I guess I wasn't real obvious, huh?
>
> Therapist: Well, sometimes it can be hard to guess how someone is feeling. Remember, we can hide our feelings. And sometimes they are not really hidden but masked because we might be feeling more than one thing. You can think about it like the weather—image a partly cloudy day that still has some sunshine.
>
> Tyiesha: Yeah.
>
> Therapist: Why would someone hide their feelings?

TYIESHA: I don't know—maybe it is not hiding but they just forget to let people know how they are feeling.

THERAPIST: Yeah—right. What other reasons?

TYIESHA: I don't know.

THERAPIST: I bet sometimes being mad at someone clouds over good feelings. For example, what if I liked what someone did, maybe they gave me a Krispy Kreme doughnut, but I was still mad at them because of something that happened earlier . . .

As can be discerned from this brief example, bringing the game into personally meaningful situations can lead to important and direct conversations about how these emotion-related concepts are relevant to the client's life.

Emotion Videos

This activity involves the therapist and client watching and discussing videos of emotional situations. A lower-tech alternative is also described.

Preparation. In advance of the activity, the therapist will need to assemble video examples and have the technology needed to show the videos to the client. There are many great examples of emotion expression that have been recorded for television and films, and with online video services becoming more and more common, accessing them easily and with limited or no cost is possible for many therapists. Assembling videos that run the gamut of feelings is important, of course. It is also a good idea to assemble videos that vary in terms of the obviousness of the emotion being depicted. If video resources are not available, an alternative is for the therapist to have some good scenes from a movie or TV show or book in mind and to describe them to the client in some detail. Note: given the variation of caregiver preferences with regard to children's viewing of entertainment, it's best to check with a caregiver before showing video snippets to a client.

This activity has the potential to teach all three skills of the module, and clip selection can be done accordingly. To follow the progression outlined in the module, therapists would aim to have the first clips show simple emotion displays, using them to teach and practice knowing feelings words and connecting feelings to body actions. Later clips would move to more complex or more ambiguous emotion displays. The final clips should depict situations in which knowledge about the person experiencing the emotion (e.g., knowledge that he is afraid of riding bikes) helps the client to identify the feeling.

Gameplay. The game is played very similarly to Feelings Detectives/Emotion Charades. Therapist and client watch a clip together (or discuss a scene) and then work together to identify the feeling or feelings expressed by the character(s) in the scene, with a focus on identifying the clues used to make that judgment.

Step 2. Rating Emotion Intensity

Overview

The goal is to introduce and practice the idea that feelings possess varied intensities and knowing the intensity of one's own and others' feelings can be helpful when coping with those feelings. The basic skill developed here cuts across a fair number of other skills-based training approaches because of the focus on ratings of problem intensity or symptom severity. In some of these treatment programs, the skill is called monitoring. For therapists who regularly use monitoring in their work, teaching Step 2 of this module will be familiar.

Teach

Why Rating Feelings Is Important

Emotions come in different intensities, like the spiciness of salsa or the difficulty levels of a video game. Knowing when one is *super* angry versus *just a little* ticked off can be really handy because it helps to know how much one will need to cope. Also, it can help to contemplate how upset one "should" be in the situation—overreaction and underreaction are both possibilities to consider. Similarly, knowing the intensity of others' emotions also helps successfully maintain relationships. For example, being able to tell that one's friend Toby is very anxious about something when one is not can help one to react more skillfully to his anxious statements. The skill can also help one anticipate future situations and thus to prepare for them. For example, if Tanya notices that she becomes very anxious when she has to go to the front of the class and give a speech, she is in a better position to prepare for the next time she gives a speech.

A key point is that feelings can be "rated" using a scale to communicate their intensity. Using numbers can help the client and therapist come to a shared understanding about just how "bad" or "good" the feeling was. Although use of a numeric scale is emphasized, the scale can be adjusted to client preference and developmental level (e.g., pictures, varying rating scales such as 0–5, 0–10, or 0–100). A number is not needed but can prove very useful in part because it permits easier comparison across events.

Practice: Activities and Games

The games listed here are particularly useful for practicing the "rating" skill, although they can be adapted for the first and third steps as well.

Rate My Last Five Feelings Game

This is a simple and fast-played game that gives clients a chance to practice the rating skill.

Preparation. No preparation is needed for this game, although it can be useful to have paper and pencil with which to record the last five feelings.

Gameplay. First, client and therapist generate a list of their last five feelings. That is, the last five feelings they experienced that they can remember. Obviously, it is not important to be literal about this. The idea is to create a list of five recent feelings. With list in hand, each person takes turns rating each one.

The game can be made more immediate by including a role play as a means to jog players' memories. Sometimes the therapist will need to provide several models before the client begins to participate actively. For particularly hesitant clients, generating a list of another person's feelings can be a good first step. A focus on others may also be useful for clients who have a difficult time with perspective taking.

Once ratings are generated for each of the last five feelings, the players then take turns talking about why each particular rating was given. For example, how did the client decide that she was a 7 out of 10? Was she paying attention to how her body felt? Did she compare the intensity of the feeling to past situations? Did she consider how important (or not) the event was to her personally? The following case example demonstrates this game. Sally is a 9-year-old girl in treatment for separation and social anxiety.

> SALLY: Well, I got really sad when I thought Herlo, our cat, was missing. She got out by accident and I couldn't find her for a real long time. That would be a 10 for me. I was really sad!
>
> THERAPIST: That sounds like a tough situation. Thanks for sharing it. Did Herlo come back?
>
> SALLY: Yeah—she came back later that night. But I was really sad and crying, crying, crying when she was gone.
>
> THERAPIST: I'm really glad she came back. It sounds like one way you knew you were really sad was you were crying. What other things did you notice that helped you know you were super sad, like a 10 on the scale?
>
> SALLY: Well, I don't know. She is *my* cat, you know, since I was little. So she is my favorite and I am hers. I would have really missed her.
>
> THERAPIST: Yeah, that's right. How we feel in our body is one way we know how big our feelings are. Another way is knowing how important something is to us.

Keep a few tips in mind here. Although tempting, one need not always push hard to get "clinically relevant" feelings and situations into the mix if the situations and feelings nominated by the client seem rather distant from the main problems that brought the client in. This is especially true early in treatment. Sometimes developing a skill can be easier outside of a context that adds stress. For example, problem solving is a technique often used for a variety of client problems. A therapist can teach problem solving to a client without specifically working on a significant problem in the client's life. Instead, a therapist can identify a simpler, less emotionally loaded problem, like how to find a lost toy. In doing so, the client learns how to use the skill, with the aim of later applying it to the more germane problems in her life.

A related tip is for therapists to use their own examples—personal or those about "another" kid—and select them to be parallel to areas of trouble/stress for the client, masking them just enough for plausibility.

As an example, imagine a 10-year-old client named Will who gets angry when he is teased on the playground. In playing the Rate My Last Five Feelings Game, let's say Will does not suggest any peer-related situations. Instead of pushing for him to generate those examples, a therapist can still find ways to discuss the situations. Two effective strategies are referencing the "back-pocket kid" and using appropriate self-disclosure. The back-pocket kid, as mentioned earlier, is an amalgamated "client" who has been through all the problems known to humankind and is based on the clinical experiences of the therapist. This kid always seems to have had a problem that comes in handy!

Self-disclosure is also a good strategy to use, provided one is always doing it for the client's benefit. For those not practiced in self-disclosure, it is generally wise to rehearse in advance before trying it "live," as good examples are hard to come by. The following examples depict both strategies in action.

THE BACK-POCKET KID

"I know a kid named Sam . . . he is a little older than you, about 12, I think, and he rides the bus to school. He told me that sometimes there is a kid on the bus who hits him with paper spitballs and that it makes him super angry. On our 0-to-10 scale, he said he gets up to an 8, really steamed! His face gets hot, and his fists clench up, and he gets this weird feeling his stomach, like it is burning or something."

SELF-DISCLOSURE

"When I was a kid, I remember one thing that really bugged me was when people called me by my middle name, except they used the short version of the name and they liked to use words that rhymed with it. My middle name is Arthur, the short version is Art, and I bet you can guess how they made fun of me. Anyway, that always made me really mad—like an 8 or 9 on our scale. It made me sad, too—like a 7 on our scale. It made my face feel hot and also made me want to hide, like I wanted to get away from everyone. Sometimes I even wanted to punch those guys. And other times, I even felt a little like I wanted to cry."

Note that in the second example, the therapist pushed the boundary of the skill by explaining that he felt more than one feeling in the situation. One can *push the boundary* with emotional awareness by (1) discussing the experience of having multiple emotions about the same event, (2) describing how a feeling rose in intensity and then fell, and (3) modeling how to use a coping strategy to change the intensity of a feeling. Each of these "boundary pushers" foreshadows a skill that could be presented later.

Ladder Game

The Ladder Game is an advanced version of the Rate My Last Five Feelings Game.

Preparation. Very little preparation is needed for this game. Index cards or paper and a pencil can be handy to write down the feeling words. It can also be useful to have the steps of the game written on an index card for reference.

Gameplay. The therapist and client work together to create a list of feelings. If an Emotion Dictionary was made earlier, those words can be used. Otherwise, a simple list of emotions is sufficient. Once the list is ready, each person takes a turn identifying a time when he or she felt each feeling. When describing the situation, role play can be used. Then an intensity rating is assigned. Next, the therapist and client work together as movie directors to imagine how to change the scene so that the feeling would "move up (or down) the ladder"—that is, how to change aspects of the situation to increase (or decrease) the intensity of the feeling. The following case example demonstrates several variations of the game and how the game can be used to teach the "rating" skill, as well as foreshadow other skills found in later modules of the book, such as emotion regulation. The client here is Chad, the 9-year-old who is thought to have ADHD. Here, he and his therapist are early in treatment. The following example comes after the therapist has explained the Ladder Game to Chad.

THERAPIST: Okay, I will go first—unless you want to?

CHAD: No. You.

THERAPIST: This goes kind of fast—are you ready? First, I pick one of the feelings. I'll go with scared. Now I'll think of a time I felt that way recently. Hmm, aha! I felt scared when I was driving and a car swerved and almost hit my car. It was pretty scary because we were on the freeway and going pretty fast. So I felt scared—my heart was pounding and I felt my body get all tense. Hmm, now, did I forget anything? *(Looks at game steps written on card.)*

CHAD: *(looking at card too)* You gotta do a rating.

THERAPIST: Oh yeah, a rating. Let me look at the scale—I would go with a 7 on that one. Anything else I need to do?

CHAD: *(looking at card again, reading)* Tell how you knew you were that rating?

THERAPIST: Right! What in my body told me how I was feeling? Well, my heart was definitely racing. And I was holding the steering wheel pretty tight. Let's see. I felt like I was ready to run a million miles or something. Lots of energy. You know that feeling?

CHAD: Yeah—maybe.

THERAPIST: Okay, next, we'll go *up* and *down* the ladder. Which way do you want to go first?

CHAD: Up. That means make it scarier, right?

THERAPIST: Right. So how would we do that?

CHAD: Well, you could have had a crash.

THERAPIST: Yikes—yep! If I'd crashed that definitely would have made it scarier. What do you think my rating would be?

CHAD: I don't know—maybe all the way to the top?

THERAPIST: I think so, yeah. A 10! Yikes! Okay, what else would make it up go up?

CHAD: I don't know.

THERAPIST: What if someone was in my car and they started yelling or getting upset?

CHAD: That would make it worse, I think. But it might make you mad, too.

THERAPIST: Great idea! And pretty complicated, too, right? I might be scared *and* mad. Two tough feelings at the same time. Not too fun. Okay, let's go down the ladder on this one. What would make it go down?

CHAD: Maybe if you were driving slower?

THERAPIST: Yeah—good one! If my speed was lower, I might not have felt so scared. Maybe knock off a point or two. Say a 5. What else?

CHAD: I don't know.

THERAPIST: Making it less scary. Hmm. What if I just saw a car almost swerve into another car, but it wasn't happening to me?

CHAD: Yeah, easier.

THERAPIST: Right. I wonder if there is anything *I* could have done to make it easier?

CHAD: Maybe you could have not driven on the freeway?

THERAPIST: Okay, right. If I had driven on a slower road, even if someone almost hit me, maybe it would have been easier?

CHAD: Maybe.

THERAPIST: Let's come up with one more. I wonder if there's anything I could say to myself that would help me feel less afraid?

CHAD: Well, you didn't have a wreck.

THERAPIST: Right, right. No wreck. That happens to me sometimes—I think of some bad thing that might happen, but when it doesn't I forget to remind myself that things turned out okay.

CHAD: Yeah—if there wasn't a wreck, then things turned out okay.

Rate the Movie/TV/Book Characters Game

The game involves showing video clips or discussing fictional scenes and then rating the characters' emotions.

Preparation. This game can draw on many forms of media, including films, TV shows, some video games, comic books, and picture books. Older children may also be able to play by recounting scenes from novels or other fictional stories, although this requires the therapist to be familiar with the book(s) in question. Video examples, of course, require certain technology and more advanced preparation.

Gameplay. The game involves therapist and client watching or hearing about the emotional scenes and then providing an emotional intensity rating for the target character(s) along with some description of *why* that rating was assigned. The game can also involve a "bonus round" that involves the client and therapist stating what their own ratings would be if they were in the situation. This helps build perspective-taking skills as well as emotion intensity rating skills.

To provide an example, three scenes from the fifth Harry Potter film, *Harry Potter and the Order of the Phoenix*, are described.

In an early scene, Harry's cousin, Dudley, and friends tease Harry. This scene is a good one for helping children recognize anger both from situational cues and also from facial and bodily cues. Obviously, the situation is one in which most children would become angry. Dudley is not just gently teasing—instead, he "goes for the jugular," mocking Harry because his parents are dead. The scene also lends itself nicely to talking about how Harry might actually also feel sad because of the losses that Dudley is mocking.

Several scenes in the film depict happiness and joy well. One in particular occurs when Neville, an apparently clumsy student and friend of Harry's, achieves great success in casting a particular spell. In addition to happiness/joy, Neville and Harry appear to experience pride, based on their facial expressions and the comments they make to each other.

A third scene depicts worry nicely. Harry's best friends, Hermione and Ron, are talking with him about the harsh (and undeserved) punishment he is receiving from a teacher named Professor Umbridge. Harry appears rather hopeless, expressing his desire to keep things to himself rather than say anything to school personnel. Both Ron and Hermione appear worried, discernible from their facial expressions and from the situational cues.

The examples provided here are just that—examples chosen to illustrate ways to identify emotion expressions in a film with which many children will be familiar.

Step 3. Expressing Emotions

Overview

Learning how (and when) to express feelings is crucial to emotion awareness and often problematic for children with mental health problems. In addition, expressing emotions is often an early step in emotion regulation, and as such, has a high degree of both interapersonal and interpersonal relevance. The sixth module in the book focuses more closely on emotional expression as it pertains to emotion regulation.

Teach

Effective Expression of Feelings Has Many Benefits

Emotion expression is not only the facial and bodily expression of emotion but also the verbal and/or written expression of feelings. Expressing feelings is important because it helps people to feel better, get along better with others (friends, family), and solve problems. Expressing feelings takes practice, just like any skill, and at first it can feel awkward and be challenging. There are several main points to cover.

Why Expression Is Important. There are many ways to express emotions. Knowing about those different ways—including how to express emotions yourself and how to recognize emotional expression in others—can help people feel better and get along with others. People express emotions to communicate with others about things that are important to them, like goals they have, or people or things they care about.

The Many Forms of Expression. People can convey feelings by using facial expressions, body language, direct verbal communication, indirect verbal communication, behaviors, and written expression. The activities and games described below emphasize the importance of "telling" feelings. In addition to covering the basic feeling–expression connections, like smiling and laughing to indicate happiness, it can also be useful for the therapist to share some personal idiosyncratic expressions to help spur the client to consider his or her own unique expression profile. As a personal example, I often share with clients that one sign I am anxious is that I feel sleepy. If I feel sleepy even though I've had plenty of sleep lately, and there is something tough coming up, that's one indication I am feeling nervous.

Hiding Feelings. Even when people hide their emotions, they are still experiencing those emotions. That feelings can be hidden makes identifying the emotions of others trickier. There are many reasons you might choose to hide feelings, and in some situations it might even be the "best" course of action (e.g., in families where expressing certain feelings is regularly punished). Thus therapists should not take the position that expressing feelings is always a virtue. Instead, therapists can emphasize that hiding (or expressing) feelings requires strategic thinking *almost every time*. Often, a client gets stuck in the "hiding" or "expressing" mode, insensitive to context. An important goal is to help clients be more aware and sensitive to their context, so that they can make good and adaptive choices about when and how to express their emotions. The worksheet **Things Are Not Always as They Seem (Handout 3)** can aid with this point; it asks clients to guess what emotion a person might experience in a given situation, and it then provides more information and asks the client to reevaluate his guess.

Feelings Can Be Expressed Even When We're Not "Trying" to Express Them. Sometimes people start to express their feelings even before they are aware they are having them. For example, a person could stamp his foot or make the "steam escaping sound" before he even "knows" he is feeling frustrated. Normalizing this phenomenon is important, as is emphasizing that as one learns more about one's own feelings, these sudden expressions can become less frequent and less intense.

Using Words for Expression. By labeling and describing feelings, people are not only expressing themselves, but are also doing two other important things: externalizing those feelings (which can make it easier for them to deal with the feelings) and communicating their feelings to others (which can help by enlisting aid). Too often, clients feel "attacked" or "overwhelmed" by feelings. By using words to express feelings (either spoken or written, but particularly in a supportive conversation with another), clients take a step toward adaptive emotion regulation. Using words can be as simple as saying, "I feel angry," although identifying the causes of the feeling represents a more advanced method.

Practice Improves Expression. With practice, people can actually get better at expressing their own feelings clearly, expressing them in ways that are not mean to others, and reading other people's expressions.

Practice: Activities and Games

The two games described here are particularly useful for practicing emotional expression, although like the earlier games, they also can be adapted to practice the first two steps.

Improv Emotions Game

This game is based on improvisational comedy, where actors improvise scenes based on information pulled from the audience.

Preparation. Index cards or slips of paper are needed as aids. Aside from that, preparation is minimal.

Gameplay. In the game, the therapist and client generate a list of emotions and write them on index cards or slips of paper. The cards are shuffled and then placed around the room. The therapist and client take turns walking to a card, reading it, and then acting out a scene that involves the feeling written on the card.

The first person to go has the "easy job," in that all he needs to do is pick up a card and then act out a brief scene depicting the feeling listed. The next person (and all players after) selects the next card and has to depict the emotion on the card in a way that fits in with the previous emotion depicted. For example, imagine the first emotion was anger, and the client pretended to be angry about the room being a mess. The second player selects a card that reads *worry.* That player then must act out a scene depicting worry that is related in some way to the first player's anger about the mess in the room. Perhaps he worries out loud, "Mom is going to be really mad about this messy room. I bet she will ground me." After each player depicts the feeling, the other player has to guess the feeling of the other person and identify any cues used to make the guess.

Paper Plate Mask Game

This game, which involves a combination of art and acting, is often a good one to use with younger children, although some older children also like it.

Preparation. Therapists will need paper plates (sheets of paper also work in a pinch) that are easy to draw and color on. Glossy plates do not work well, so luckily the less expensive plates are often the best. In addition, the game involves the use of five emotional scenarios (examples provided below) in which a person might experience one emotion on the inside while expressing another emotion outwardly. Although these scenarios can be created during the session, it is useful to have them written out in advance. These are certainly not the only nor are they necessarily the best examples. Always look for places to tailor examples to the client's own situation.

Scenario 1: You are on the bus going to school after your mom just yelled at you a lot to hurry up getting ready.

Scenario 2: You just received your test back and you got an A. You notice that your best friend got a D.

Scenario 3: You are at the movies with a group of friends. The movie you are seeing is really scary.

Scenario 4: You are in class and a story your teacher was reading reminded you of your dog who died last year.

Scenario 5: On the playground, a kid starts to tease you about your clothes or hair.

Gameplay. The object of the game is to make paper plate masks for different scenarios. Therapist and client take turns selecting one scenario randomly and then drawing faces on the plates to reflect feelings. One side of the plate—the outer—represents what the person would show the world, and the other side—the inner—represents how the person really feels. After making a plate for each scenario, the therapist and client take turns sharing what they made and why they made it the way they did.

The paper plate game allows not only for clear depiction of emotion facial expressions but also permits the beginning of a discussion of the "strategies" involved in hiding emotion expression. The therapist can share, for example, how he might hide feelings of embarrassment from being teased (Scenario 5) by thinking of something funny or looking at a friend. As clients become comfortable with self-disclosure, the game also creates opportunities for the therapist to learn about which feelings the client prefers to keep hidden.

Alternate Version 1: Expansion. A twist on the Paper Plate Mask Game that leads to potentially greater understanding of how the client expresses and hides feelings involves using the same scenario multiple times, each time altering one or two variables. Take Scenario 1 from above, in which the child was yelled at by his or her mother while getting ready for school and is now on the school bus. The therapist could change (1) mother to father, (2) yelling to crying, (3) yelling to worrying, (4) bus to car ride with mother, (5) bus to carpool with friends, and so on. Here, the game within a game becomes the therapist's quest to test the limits of the client's understanding of emotion expression and to generate hypotheses for the family dynamics involved in creating and supporting these expressions. In this way, the game serves as another tool to facilitate the functional analysis described in Chapter 4.

Alternate Version 2: Words. Another version of the game involves a "next step" in which the client (and therapist) tells *with whom* and *how* he or she would share the hidden feelings and then role-play doing just that. It is generally a good practice to model this for clients first; thus therapists are encouraged to collect examples from their own lives.

Feelings, Feelings, Everywhere!

A. Feelings I have had recently

1. _____

2. _____

3. _____

4. _____

5. _____

B. Feelings someone in my family had recently

1. _____

2. _____

3. _____

4. _____

5. _____

C. Other feeling words I have heard people say

1. _____

2. _____

3. _____

4. _____

5. _____

Feelings and Our Bodies

Match the feeling wotrds on the left to the body feelings on the right. Feel free to add emotions and body feelings. Each emotion can have more than one body feeling.

EMOTIONS	BODY FEELINGS
1. Anger	A. <u>Funny feelings in my stomach</u>
2. Happiness	B. <u>Hot feelings in my face</u>
3. Worry	C. <u>My head aches</u>
4. Excitement	D. <u>My hands are shaking</u>
5. Fear	E. <u>I am crying</u>
6. Sadness	F. <u>My fists are clenched</u>
7. _____	G. <u>I am smiling</u>
8. _____	H. _____
9. _____	I. _____
10. _____	J. _____
11. _____	K. _____

Things Are Not Always as They Seem

Sometimes we can't know how someone is feeling unless we know something about that person. Try to guess what feeling each kid would feel in these situations.

Write down an emotion for each situation before moving on to the next one.

1. Darrius's neighbor just got a new dog that really likes kids.

   _____

2. Darrius's neighbor just got a new dog that really likes kids, but Darrius was once bitten by a dog.

   _____

3. Reena has to give a big speech tomorrow in front of her entire school.

   _____

4. Reena has to give a big speech tomorrow in front of her entire school, and Reena loves to give speeches.

   _____

5. Jenny got an A on her math test.

   _____

6. Jenny got an A on her math test, but she cheated on it.

   _____

MODULE 2

Emotion Understanding Skills

Emotion awareness, the focus of the previous module, is one of the earliest acquired emotional competence skills. Arguably, emotion understanding comes next. Emotion understanding is a child's *knowledge* about emotions: how they "feel," what causes them, how they "work," and how they can be hidden or changed. The word *knowledge* is emphasized because emotion understanding is a matter of knowing rather than doing. Emotion-related "doing" is the focus of the modules on empathy and emotion regulation.

WHEN TO USE THIS MODULE

This module is designed for use when a major contributor to a client's difficulties is the lack of knowledge about emotions and is designed to be a next developmental step after emotion awareness—that is, knowing that one is experiencing an emotion, being aware of the intensity of that feeling, and having the capability to express the feeling. Clients who may benefit the most from this module are those with a limited understanding of at least one of the following emotion-related concepts: (1) emotions are caused or triggered by both environmental and internal events, (2) more than one feeling can occur at a time, (3) specific feelings affect the body in specific ways, or (4) feelings can be hidden or changed.

OBJECTIVES

The objectives for this module are to teach and practice a set of four emotion concepts to build understanding of them as a foundation for other emotion-related skills, such as empathy and emotion regulation.

1. **Emotion triggers.** Emotions can be caused by both environmental and internal events.
2. **Multiple emotions.** People can experience more than one feeling at the same time.
3. **Emotions affect our bodies.** Different emotions have different effects on people's bodies.
4. **Emotions can be hidden (or changed).** People can hide or change their emotions; what they show the world is not necessarily what they feel. The focus of this module will be on hiding emotions; later modules will place greater emphasis on the fact that they can be changed.

PROCEDURES
Step 1. Triggering Feelings

Overview

When asked, "Why are you angry?" a client might respond, "She tripped me" or "The game is broken." Understanding these external triggers is a developmentally early step and an important one. But sometimes the equally important triggers are *inside* the client: a belief he has, a value he holds dearly, a fear he has hidden. These internal cues are only recognized later in development and are, understandably, harder to come by.

Teach

What Triggers Feelings

The basic concept here is simple. Feelings occur in response to *events*, which may be external (like success in a sporting match or in the classroom, or disappointment in either venue) or internal (related to the client's beliefs, aspirations, and preferences). This key teaching point is not so hard to make. Clients often readily understand that feelings happen in response to events, and they will often quickly describe several examples of times when they experienced some event and then had a feeling in response. But most young children's initial understanding of how feelings are triggered represents only part of the story. The harder knowledge to come by is the fact that how a client thinks about a situation often influences her feelings as much as or more than the situation itself. The main teaching point here can be easily stated, yet understanding is more challenging to confirm, and so practicing is often a focus for this step. Fortunately, there are several creative ways to convey the main idea contained in Step 1.

Generating a list of reasons for feelings can be an easy way to get the topic introduced, and the **Feelings and Triggers** worksheet (**Handout 1**) is one way to generate and organize this list. Therapists may find it useful to provide their own examples, particularly with regard to internal triggers. Calculated self-disclosure is one effective strategy, but examples abound in media as well. In the therapy excerpt below, a therapist uses self-disclosure to convey the point that the causes of feelings can sometimes be not-so-obvious and also hidden to observers. The client, Emma, is an 11-year-old with lots of worries and a likely ADHD diagnosis, predominantly inattentive subtype.

THERAPIST: I want to tell you a little story. Once upon a time, when I was about 12 years old, my family decided to go to a lake near our house with another family during the summer. We were going to camp near the lake and then do water sports like swimming and fishing. Do you ever do stuff like that with your family?

EMMA: Yeah, we go to the river sometimes.

THERAPIST: Same kind of thing, I think. So how do you think I would feel about this trip?

EMMA: Hmm, I don't know. Good, I guess. I mean, that sounds pretty fun.

THERAPIST: Right! Good. So the triggers for my feelings that we can see are fun activities, right? How could we get more information to help us guess how I might feel?

EMMA: Um, I don't know. We could ask you?

THERAPIST: That would be a good way to do it, for sure! What if we couldn't ask, though, and we had to look for clues for how I would feel? What clues would there be?

EMMA: Well, hmm. Maybe if we knew who was going with you?

THERAPIST: Good one! Right! So I can tell you that the family coming with us had a boy about my age . . . and I liked him. He was nice and kind of cute.

EMMA: Oh, that can be kind of, um . . .

THERAPIST: Tricky?

EMMA: Yeah—like, depends on what he thinks about you?

THERAPIST: Right! And I was worried it would be awkward because of my folks being around. They could be sorta . . .

EMMA: Embarrassing—yeah, I know about that.

THERAPIST: Right! So the activities sound like I would be happy, but having this boy there makes it a little more complicated. I might feel shy or worried or even anxious. And one more thing. What if I told you I didn't know how to swim?

EMMA: Oh, really? That would be embarrassing, too.

THERAPIST: I know. I was afraid the boy and his family would find out I was a terrible swimmer and that would be so embarrassing. I was really pretty stressed about it.

EMMA: Yeah, I had this friend and she didn't know how to swim and she wouldn't ever come to the river with us.

THERAPIST: It was tough for sure. So, knowing all of that, how do you think I was feeling about the trip?

EMMA: Well, I guess maybe kind of worried, like you said. And also maybe even worse than that, like stressed.

THERAPIST: What about excited?

EMMA: Hmm, I don't know. Maybe. Why would you be excited?

THERAPIST: Well, there is that feeling you get when you like a boy. That can be nice. So even though I was worried and stressed, I was also kind of excited.

This excerpt nicely shows how to use calculated self-disclosure to model how feelings are caused by both internal and external triggers. Notice, too, how the therapist also demonstrates the second step of the module—that one situation can cause more than one feeling.

Practice: Activities and Games

The following two games can be used to teach and practice the notion that feelings are triggered.

Trigger Card Game

Preparation. This game requires a set of feeling cards. These can be index cards with a feeling word written on each one. The feelings on the cards can be generated by the client and therapist in the meeting or else created before the session.

Gameplay. In the game, the first player draws a card and places it face up between the players. The player reads the card and provides an example of a trigger for that feeling (from his or her own life or from anyone else's life). The next player lists another trigger for the same feeling. Play continues for four rounds (i.e., eight total triggers) or until one of the players runs out of ideas for triggers (whichever comes first). Scores are assigned as follows: one point for each external trigger, two points for each internal trigger, and three points for personal triggers (i.e., triggers that are true for oneself). The player with the highest point total for the card draws the next card. Play proceeds until one player scores a set number of points (e.g., 30, 50, 100) or until the feeling cards run out.

Alternate Version 1: Charades. For each card, the player creates a charades-like scene that includes one or more triggers for the feeling. The other player has to guess the feeling and the trigger(s) involved. Points can be awarded as follows: The player earns 2 points for guessing the emotion correctly on the first guess, 1 point for guessing on the second or third guess, and no points for taking more than three guesses. Points for triggers are awarded in the same way as described earlier, with players earning points for both acting out triggers as well as guessing them correctly.

Alternate Version 2: Art. Instead of a game, an artistic medium can be used to convey triggers. For example, the therapist and client could create a book that depicts, either in pictures or words, a set of feelings and their triggers. Similarly, the therapist and client could make a video that does the same thing. Or paint a picture or create a sculpture from modeling clay that accomplishes the task.

Alternate Version 3: Movies. Therapists with access to clips from movies or TV shows that depict emotion scenes can use these instead of cards. The players would take turns generating the triggers for the character's emotions. Carefully chosen media clips can even show a continuation or follow-up to earlier clips that provide more information that changes the perception of the trigger.

Inside/Outside Game

This is a simpler game that includes a physical activity element and thus may be a good one for younger and more active clients.

Preparation. This game requires two distinct physical spaces. These can be delineated in any of a number of ways, including chalk, yarn, differing floor or rug colors, or specific objects, like a couch or table. The two spaces should be relatively distant from each other, such that to get from one to the other, one needs to cover a few yards (more can be better, so outside spaces or a gymnasium can work well). One of the spaces should be labeled *inside* and the other *outside*. In a tight space or with limited materials on hand, one can even just delineate one space the inside and then let the remaining space be *outside*; even opposite walls of room work. The objective here is to make two distinct locations.

Before playing, a set of cards describing people in different emotional situations is needed. Some examples follow.

Scenario 1: Taya is in school and starts feeling very anxious.

Scenario 2: Walking home from school, Scott starts to feel really sad.

Scenario 3: In his room at home, Antwan becomes very angry.

Scenario 4: At the park, Mei-Yi becomes very happy.

Note how simple these prompts are. It is best to avoid creating prompts with obvious triggers. Note, too, that one need not even create these prompts in advance, as they can be created as the game proceeds.

Gameplay. To begin the game, the players stand in a location that is neither INSIDE or OUTSIDE. One of the players reads a scenario. Players then take turns saying a trigger for the emotion in the situation. After each trigger is offered, the player stating the trigger indicates whether it is something external or internal by running to the correct location. For each situation, the goal is to identify at least four different triggers, including at least one internal trigger.

The game can also be played in a competitive way. After each trigger, all players race to the correct space. Award one point to the first person to make it to the correct space. The first person to 10 points wins. Although the game is designed to be fast paced, in between triggers the therapist is encouraged to teach and help the client to generalize to situations that pertain directly to the client. For example, when considering reasons why Taya is nervous about school, one can recall that the client was nervous once about going to school, which may lead into a conversation about that event.

Step 2. Experiencing Multiple Emotions at the Same Time

Overview

One of the most complicating and remarkable facts about the emotional lives of humans is the simultaneous experience of multiple emotions. The fact that humans do have more than one feeling at a time seems obvious to most therapists, but the fact escapes children (and some adults) for many years of their lives. Developing this knowledge starts with a rather simple understanding: "I can have more than one feeling at the same time when each feeling is related to a different target." For example, Lucille can feel upset about losing a toy but also excited about the upcoming field trip at school. Next, children come to understand that they can feel more than one feeling about the same target, so long as those feelings are relatively similar in content. For example, Lucille can feel both happy and excited about an upcoming event. Finally, children come to understand that it is possible to have opposite or discordant emotions about the same target at the same time. For example, Lucille can feel angry at her mother, yet also love her at the same time. Developmental science indicates that children tend to reach these understandings in early elementary school and that younger children will deny that feeling more than one thing at the same time is possible.

Teach

People Sometimes Have More Than One Feeling at the Same Time

Understanding the concept of multiple emotions is important for a few reasons. First, knowing that one can experience multiple emotions simultaneously helps to facilitate emotion regulation. This is particularly true when one experiences multiple feelings about the same target. For example, Lucille may be excited and anxious about an upcoming event. Knowing that she has both feelings may help her to cope better, as the ways to cope with excitement differ from those for anxiety.

Second, relationships are often a context for multiple emotions, and knowing that one can feel angry with and yet still love (or like) significant others is important as it may help one better maintain those relationships.

A simple and effective way to help clients understand these important concepts is by providing examples. For instance, one can describe a time when something good happens to someone we love, but the "good" thing means that the person moves away—such as getting into college or getting a new job. On one hand, one feels happy for the person; on the other hand, one is sad to be "losing" the friend. These mixed or multiple feelings are normal but can be confusing. It can be hard to know how to behave when one experiences apparently contradictory feelings.

Sometimes, too, feelings can come one after the other in quick succession. This can happen in many ways, but one example clients can often relate to is the "scared to angry" progression. The following brief story is one example.

Imagine you are sitting at your desk in school, reading quietly or day-dreaming. Suddenly, your friend claps her hands loudly in your ears, startling you. You suddenly feel really scared—like you are going to jump out of your skin! Next, though, you might feel a rush of feelings, including anger, and you snap at your friend, "What's the big idea?" Maybe you even accompany the snappy remark with a shove.

Yet another way to describe this to clients is to explain that feelings happen in a complex ways, more like cars on a busy freeway than cars passing through a tollbooth. Feelings happen at all sorts of speeds. Also, sometimes they are spaced out like a highway with almost no traffic. Other times they are packed in together, like a traffic jam.

Finally, it is also important to explain that when people have more than one feeling at the same time, sometimes that makes things confusing because the feelings affect each other. For example, imagine that Darrius is best friends with Harold and that both tried out for the school play. They are both looking at the list of students who received parts, and Darrius is on the list but Harold is not. Darrius is thrilled at first to see his name, but when he doesn't see Harold's, and then sees Harold's face, Darrius's excitement about making it is changed by his disappointment that Harold did not make it.

As always, these teaching examples can be supplemented with or replaced by the game described next.

Practice: Activities and Games

This section of the module contains a game that can be used to teach and practice the notion that people sometimes feel more than one feeling at once.

Emotional Emmy Game

Preparation. Before playing, the therapist will need to create a deck of emotion cards that list different feelings. The cards can simply have the emotion words on them or they can have the word along with a picture, similar to the commonly found wall posters that ask the question: "How are you feeling today?" The deck should have at least 30 cards, and there should be multiple occurrences of the same feelings. Index cards work great, and therapists may want to laminate their decks, as they will hold up better. There are two variations of Emotional Emmy described here, and readers are encouraged to create their own variations.

Gameplay. There are two primary variations of the game. In the first, the deck is shuffled and then placed face down in the center of the playing area. The first player selects the top two cards and places shows them to the other player(s). The first player then tells a story about a character named Emotional Emmy; the story must involve Emmy experiencing *both* emotions listed on the cards at the same time. Play alternates and ends when a player reaches 20 points, with points awarded by the other players as follows:

1 point	Story involves Emmy experiencing at least one of the emotions on the cards.
3 points	Story involves Emmy experiencing both emotions on the cards.
4 points	Story involves Emmy experiencing both emotions on the cards at the same time.
5 points	Story involves Emmy experiencing both emotions on the cards at the same time about the same target.

Alternate Version: Challenge. Here, the deck is shuffled and 10 cards are dealt to each player, face down. The players then look at their cards, and the first player lays down any card of his choosing face-up on the table. The other player then plays any one of her cards, challenging the first play to create an Emmy story that combines these two emotions. Scoring follows the same procedure detailed above.

Step 3. Feeling the Effects of Different Emotions on Our Bodies

Overview

Feelings are associated with physiological signals. Some signals are specific to one or a few feelings, whereas others are associated with many feelings. Though this learning point is also relevant for emotional awareness, it is discussed in this module because knowing the physiological feelings represents an important understanding and advanced building block compared to emotional awareness.

Teach

The Physiology of Different Emotions

Because the physiological reactions associated with specific emotions differ, it can be useful to discuss at least the following four emotions with most clients: fear/anxiety/worry, sadness, anger, and happiness.

Fear/Anxiety/Worry. There are a number of points to make about the physiological signals relevant to fear, anxiety, and worry. Therapists can be selective when choosing which points seem most relevant to a particular client (and some points may be overly complicated for younger clients). However, when in doubt, making each point may be worth the effort. Each one is quite simple and each one is an extension of others. Thus there is not much additional time required to cover all ten points versus, say, just six.

1. **Anxiety is normal.** The human body was designed to experience fear and anxiety and part of the design was to make the feelings *strong* and *uncomfortable* so that people would take immediate action.
2. **Anxiety is experienced in physiology.** There are common ways of experiencing anxious feelings including: (a) cardiac (e.g., heart racing); (b) pulmonary (e.g., heavy breathing); (c) gastrointestinal (e.g., butterflies in the stomach); (d) bodily tension (e.g., headaches); (e) hand/foot temperature dysregulation (e.g., feeling cold hands, sweating); (f) agitation (e.g., trembling); and (g) dry mouth.
3. **Some anxious bodily feelings are similar to other, nonanxious feelings.** Some of the signals for anxiety are also signals for other feelings, including excitement and illness. For example, some people use the word *anxious* when describing their anticipation of an upcoming event about which they are excited, as in "I am anxious to start playing this game." The bodily feelings may be quite similar here, but the feeling is perhaps better described as eagerness, unless fear is also being experienced. Also, some bodily feelings that people associate with anxiety can be signs of illness, such as a stomachache.
4. **Anxiety affects people's thinking.** When feeling anxious or fearful, people tend to exaggerate threat, anticipate many more bad possible futures than are likely, and prefer solutions that involve avoidance. Some call this *emotional reasoning,* and it can lead to problematic choices.
5. **The fight-or-flight system.** Many bodily anxiety reactions are part of what is called the fight-or-flight system (FFS), which involves intense arousal

of what is called the sympathetic nervous system. Some clients may enjoy learning more about this by seeing diagrams of the sympathetic nervous system that depict the various organs and muscles systems activated by the FFS. The FFS is a helpful adaptation in situations involving real danger, but when activated in non-life-threatening situations the FFS can lead to distressing and problematic experiences, including panic attacks and behavioral avoidance. Knowing the difference between real and false FFS alarms is an important part of managing anxiety.

6. **The "Be Vigilant" System.** There is another part of the nervous system called the behavioral inhibition system (BIS) that is helpful in situations where sensing and evaluating potential dangers is paramount. The BIS helps the body become quiet (but not relaxed) so that one can be vigilant for threat. The BIS also primes the FFS for action. For example, therapists can ask a client to imagine herself reading quietly and then imagine that she hears an unfamiliar noise. What would happen? Perhaps the client would stop reading and her body would suddenly be on a quiet alert. However, just as the FFS can have false alarms, so too can our BIS become active when it's not really needed. The BIS may be associated with worrying as well as hypervigilance.

7. **Anxiety cannot be turned off quickly.** The body's experience of anxiety is not like a light switch that can be turned on and off at will. Instead, it is more like a wagon on a flat surface. Once the wagon is given a push, it keeps rolling for a while before eventually stopping (unless someone pushes the wagon again). In the same way, anxious feelings eventually subside on their own.

8. **Anxiety is fun for some, less fun for others.** Although many people experience bodily anxiety signals as uncomfortable, some enjoy the feelings and seek them out (e.g., scary movies, bungee jumping). Other people think that anxiety, worry, and stress are necessary for success.

9. **Anxiety is rarely harmful.** Unless one has certain medical conditions, the body's anxiety signals are not harmful (although they may be uncomfortable).

10. **Noticing anxiety signs helps people to cope.** Recognizing anxiety signals is a first step in coping with those feelings.

Sadness. There are six main points to make about sadness, depression, and the physiological signals relevant to sadness.

1. **Sadness is normal.** Sadness is a feeling that all people experience, especially when something bad happens, like a loss.
2. **Sadness has many physiological effects.** People's sadness-related bodily feelings are very diverse.

- Some people's bodies react to sadness in ways one can readily understand: crying, head down, hands held to head, curling up in a ball.
- When other people get sad, the reaction is more like grouchiness and anger.

3. **Sadness and depression are not the same.** Sadness and depression are similar but not the same thing. Everyone feels sad sometimes, and people may even call those feelings "being depressed." But there is also a feeling known as depression that is a longer-lasting and more severe version of sadness.

4. **Sadness goes away over time, often with effort.** Like anxiety, both sadness and depression will go away over time. However, a big difference between anxiety and sadness/depression is that anxiety tends to go away a lot more quickly. Sad or depressed feelings can sometimes linger for hours, days, and even weeks. While doing "nothing" about some feelings, like anxiety or anger, can be an effective way to cope in some instances, doing "nothing" for depression is usually a bad idea.

5. **Sadness has many symptoms.** Sadness and depression are associated with a number of physiological, behavioral, and cognitive experiences, including:
   - **Sleep problems.** Some will feel very tired and want to sleep a lot, whereas others will have lots of trouble falling or staying asleep.
   - **Appetite problems.** Some will lose their appetites, whereas others will be hungry or want to eat a lot more than is normal.
   - **Energy problems.** Some feel very low levels of energy and/or experience a feeling of lethargy. Others feel too much energy and the need to move around (also called psychomotor agitation).
   - **Concentration problems.** Some who are feeling depressed have trouble focusing, sometimes because they are thinking about situations that increase their sad feelings.
   - **Negative thinking.** Sadness often produces something called "stinking thinking," which means focusing on the negative, remembering the worst of past experiences, and anticipating negative experiences to come. When one is thinking negatively, one may not see the wisdom of someone who says, "Hey, you're not thinking too clearly about this right now."

6. **Sadness may be related to some brain chemical changes.** Therapists can discuss how brain chemicals called neurotransmitters are involved in moods; this point is probably relevant only to older children and/or those who show an interest in scientific discussions. Most readers will be familiar with the serotonin hypothesis. In short, there are really two distinct hypotheses about serotonin: (a) a lack of serotonin in the brain is a proximate cause of depression, and (b) there is a biological vulnerability in some individuals that leads to lower serotonergic activity in the brain, which in turn leads to increased risk for depression. Knowing that depression and sadness may be partly related to brain chemicals can be a difficult concept

to communicate, but for some children, particularly those with long family histories of depression, the effort is likely to be warranted.

A few points to consider when discussing the serotonin hypothesis with children:

First, the idea that there is a brain chemical deficit associated with depression is a *hypothesis.* In other words, the evidence supporting this idea is not completely solid. So by talking about brain chemicals, the therapist should be clear that he is not implying the client has a brain chemical problem and he is not saying that medication is needed to solve the problem. Instead, the brain chemical idea is used to talk about how feelings are related to changes in our brain. Changes in our brain are not directly open to manipulation—that is, one cannot make immediate changes to one's brain chemicals and have that translate to immediate changes in how one feels. Instead, one can do or think things and then observe how those thoughts or actions affect one's feelings. For sadness, a therapist can talk about how it is important for each person to know what thoughts and actions help him to feel happier when he is feeling sad.

Second, a discussion about brain chemicals can start a conversation about temperament, the unique biological "blueprint" everyone has. People get to decide some things about how they will to grow and develop, but some of the framework is already there. The unique way that each person's brain chemistry works may be part of that framework. That is, if the client tends to get sad and depressed, it might partly related to the way her brain chemicals work. Knowing that may help her because if she knows her tendencies, she may be able to better marshal the resources needed to cope.

Third, the therapist can also talk about how there is scientific evidence that behaviors and thoughts affect brain chemicals. This point can help to instill hope. It is important and useful for the client to know that she can do things to change her emotions and the brain chemicals associated with them and that there is scientific evidence demonstrating that it's possible.

One final reason to discuss brain chemicals is because some clients are already taking psychotropic medicines. It is good for clients to know that their therapists know something about medicine and brain chemicals and that that topic can be discussed if they have questions.

Anger. As with the other feelings, there are several points to make about the physiological experiences related to anger.

1. **Anger is normal.** As with all feelings, anger is not an enemy; it is a normal and expectable human experience. Anger usually tells people that something important to them is threatened in some way, or that their desire to reach a certain goal has been frustrated. Also, on a positive note, anger can stimulate assertiveness and persistence.

2. **Anger has physiological signs.** Anger is associated with a number of physiological reactions similar to those experienced with anxiety: heart rate increase, breathing rate increase, and bodily tension. One reason for the overlap is due to the FFS involvement in anger. An interesting way to connect these two feelings is to ask if clients know someone who seems angry when they are frightened. Such a situation is also a good example of how we can experience more than one feeling at the same time.

3. **Anger makes people want to act quickly.** Like anxiety, anger creates a strong desire to act immediately. This is in contrast to sadness and depression, which generally lead to a desire for inactivity.

4. **Acting on anger can lead to poor choices.** Anger, like anxiety and sadness, often impedes a person's ability to make optimal choices. Because there is often a strong push to act quickly and aggressively, therapists can encourage clients to cultivate using anger as a trigger for slowing down and not acting. This topic is covered in more depth in the emotion regulation modules. The educational point here is similar to that of anxiety insofar as the therapist's message is often: "When we feel angry, often we do well to pause and *not* act despite our strong inclination toward action."

5. **There are ways to cope with anger.** Anger's *heat* lends itself well to direct physiological coping in addition to emotional expression. Talking can help (see Module 6, Emotion Regulation Skills III: Expression Skills), as can engaging in physical activities (e.g., going on a run, see Module 5, Emotion Regulation Skills II: Mastery).

Happiness. Most clients do not have trouble managing their happiness, so it may seem unusual to spend time discussing it. But just like in parent training approaches, when there is a focus on the positive opposite of the behaviors one is trying to reduce, sometimes with "emotion education," knowledge about the feelings one would like to see increase can be helpful. There are four general points to be made about happiness.

1. **Happiness is not the same as "not feeling bad."** Happiness should not be confused with the absence of unwanted feelings like sadness, anxiety, or anger. People generally experience happiness when they are involved in an activity that brings them pleasure and/or when they are in the midst of achieving their goals. With some clients it may be good to help them recall times when they were happy and clarify how they knew the time was well spent. Unfortunately, for many clients, happy times are easily forgotten amid a lot of difficult times.

2. **Happiness has many physiological signs.** Happiness is experienced in the body in a variety of ways, including warm and buoyant feelings in the core, laughter, and a fascinating ability to ignore unpleasant or uncomfortable

feelings in one's body and to overlook memories and events that are counter to one's current feeling of happiness.

3. **Happiness is sometimes related to safety.** For clients with eager minds, therapists can make the point that other animals appear happy (and playful) when they are safe from dangers. That is, when one thinks about happiness from an evolutionary or survival-of-the-fittest perspective, one can recognize that feeling safe is related to feeling happy.

4. **Faking happiness can sometimes create happiness.** Finally, it is often interesting to let clients know there is scientific evidence suggesting that people who force themselves to smile actually experience happiness. That is, there is an apparent feedback loop between facial muscles and the brain such that when the brain catches the face smiling, the brain says, "Oh, I must be happy."

Practice: Activities and Games

The following game can be used to teach and practice the different physiological experiences associated with various feelings.

Body Signals Game

For all four of these feelings (and many more that one might consider with clients), the Body Signals game can be a good teaching tool.

Preparation. This game can be played with no advanced setup, although some therapists may prefer to take 10 minutes to prepare a list of emotion-eliciting situations. One way to do this is create a deck of cards with a single situation written on each card. There are a number of examples listed here.

Scenario 1: You are a new student in a school. In math class, the teacher calls on you to give an answer. You are afraid that your guess will be wrong and the other kids will laugh.

Scenario 2: Your mother is usually home by 5 P.M. but today it is 5:20 P.M. and she has not called you. You have called her cell phone but she is not answering. You are afraid that something bad has happened.

Scenario 3: You are babysitting and the kids are asleep. The house seems very quiet and you hear a weird noise in the backyard. You suddenly feel very scared.

Scenario 4: You are lying in bed the night before a big science test. You have studied hard for a few days now, but your mind is racing with worries about the test and the possible things that could go wrong.

Scenario 5: Your best friend has not texted or called you back, even though you two always text each other back right away. You start to worry that she is not your friend anymore, or worse yet, something bad has happened to her.

Scenario 6: You just read on the Internet about a new disease with symptoms like headache, dizziness, and a skin rash. You read that the disease is apparently caused by water-borne bacteria. You start worrying that you will get the disease because you recently drank funny-tasting water at a restaurant.

Scenario 7: Your best friend for the last 3 years is going to move out of state this summer.

Scenario 8: Your pet, who was very old, had to be put to sleep at the vet's office today. You just got home from school and your mom (or dad) confirmed that your pet is dead now.

Scenario 9: Your boyfriend/girlfriend broke up with you today after school.

Scenario 10: Your sibling went into your room today without your permission and accidentally broke one of your favorite possessions.

Scenario 11: Your parents are punishing you for having broken a house rule, and part of the punishment is that you are grounded and will miss a sleepover at your friend's house.

Scenario 12: You have been working on a school project for a few weeks, and the night before it is due you notice that the computer file you had saved is missing work you had done a few days ago. You realize that you must have forgotten to save the work from that day.

Scenario 13: You receive your report card and your grades are even better than you had hoped. You know your parents will be proud.

Scenario 14: It is Friday right before a school vacation and you have no homework to do during the break.

Scenario 15: You are having a few friends over after school and you have a new game to share with them that you know they will love.

Gameplay. The deck is shuffled and placed face down in the center of the playing area. The first player selects the top card and places it face up. The player then lists as many body signals as he can that would be associated with the scenario. For each signal listed, the other player(s) vote either "yes" or "no," signifying whether the player(s) agree that the body signal is correctly associated with the feeling. For each "yes," the player receives one point. Play alternates until one player reaches 20 points or until the card pile is exhausted.

Step 4. Hiding (and Changing) Emotions

Overview

Children learn to hide their feelings at a young age, with one of the first demonstrations of this knowledge often being what are called *display rules*. These are unwritten social rules concerning when to express (and when not to express) certain untoward feelings, with the classic example being the feeling expressed in receipt of the unwanted gift from a relative who is watching your reaction. Although the experienced emotion may be disappointment, sadness, or even anger, the expressed emotion is supposed to be happiness or gratitude. That is, one is supposed to hide one's disappointment. Many preschool children possess this capacity. *Emotional dissemblance*, as hiding one's true emotions is sometimes called, becomes more sophisticated with age, such that middle school–age children can provide detailed descriptions of contexts in which they would or would not express their emotions.

Teach

Hiding Feelings

Hiding our emotions has social benefits, and knowledge about how and why people hide their feelings is an important component of emotional competence. There are a few relevant teaching points to make.

One's Expression ≠ One's Experience. It's a simple point, but *the* primary take-home message here is that one does not have to express every feeling one experiences. In fact, there are times when expressing one's true feelings could have undesired consequences.

Others' Expression ≠ Others' Experience. This is a crucial point for emotional competence and thus social competence; accurately reading and responding to others' emotions is a critical component of social interaction.

Why Would Someone Hide His/Her Feelings? Here there are myriad reasons to consider, and the game described later can be used to illustrate this point.

How Would Someone Hide His/Her Feelings? Similar to the *why* question, the *how* of hiding feelings includes a diverse set of responses. The game described later also provides a means to practice this skill. Provided here is a list of different ways to hide one's feelings.

SAMPLE STRATEGIES FOR HOW TO HIDE FEELINGS

Fake it. This strategy is the simplest—just fake a different feeling.

Stay quiet. There are many times when saying little can be a way to keep feelings hidden.

Distract others. Verbal or physical distraction can be an effective way to hide feelings; if others are not paying attention to the person, then even if that person's feelings are showing, people will be less likely to notice.

Hide Feelings Rarely and Strategically. A final but important point: hiding feelings is sometimes socially important but is not generally a positive or healthy way to deal with feelings on a regular basis. Indeed, there is some evidence that hiding feelings often has negative effects on mental and physical health. Thus the tenor of this discussion should center on hiding feelings temporarily and in select situations. For clients who struggle to express their feelings at all and are more prone to hiding (a.k.a. *stuffing*) their feelings, the Emotion Regulation Skills III: Expression Skills module (Module 6) may be an important one to consider. Below is a sample of some situations in which hiding feelings may be helpful, at least temporarily.

WHEN HIDING FEELINGS MAY BE A GOOD IDEA

When expressing feelings will create social unease. This is the classic situation for hiding feelings: when expressing one's feelings will cause more damage than not expressing them. For example, supporting a friend in his choice even when you don't agree with or like the choice.

When the feeling may be temporary. Sometimes it is worth reminding clients that feelings are often temporary and fleeting. Expressing *every* feeling may not be the best option. Sometimes, older clients who watch reality TV shows will appreciate the wisdom of this idea, and the therapist can encourage conversation about how "overexpression" has affected particular individuals on those programs. It may be useful for therapists to have a few personal examples of their own temporary feelings ready to share.

Unsafe situations. In some situations, showing your true feelings may actually make things more dangerous, like when you show fear or hurt feelings to a bully.

Practice: Activities and Games

This section of the module contains a game that can be used to teach and practice the skill of hiding feelings.

Hiding Feelings Card Game

This game involves a combination of conversation and role play.

Preparation. The game requires a set of cards with emotional situations written on them. Index cards work well. The situations should involve characters that will be likely to hide their feelings. A few sample situations are provided here. Having a deck of about 10 cards makes for good play.

Scenario 1: Your elderly aunt gave you a present for your birthday that you don't like. She is smiling at you as you open it. You feel disappointed.

Scenario 2: One of the bullies in your school is harassing another kid and sees you watching. He shouts over to you, "What are you looking at?" You feel scared.

Scenario 3: You just struck out in your baseball game and are returning to the dugout, your teammates looking at you. You feel sad and embarrassed.

Scenario 4: You are in the 10th grade. Your locker is next to a boy/girl you think is cute but whom you don't know very well yet. He/she is walking up to the locker and you feel really nervous.

Scenario 5: Your teacher just blamed you for having done something you did not do. You feel angry.

Scenario 6: You and your friend were both vying for the lead role in the school play. Your friend was just selected for the role. You feel sad and jealous.

Gameplay. After shuffling the deck, the cards are placed face down. Players then take turns drawing a card. There are three phases of the game. In the first phase, the player reads the card and both players discuss the situation, focusing on whether hiding feelings would be a good idea—and if so, how they would do it. The second phase of the game involves the player who drew the card acting out the scene, often with the help of the other player(s), either hiding or not hiding the feeling(s), based on the discussion. The final phase of the game involves the player doing the opposite of his first choice. In other words, if in the first role play the player did hide his feelings, in the second role play he does *not* hide them.

For those clients who like to play games with scoring, the other players can rate how well the player hid his feelings on a scale of 1–5, with 5 being superior and 1 being terrible. The first player to 20 points wins.

The excerpt below provides an example of a therapist working through the first phase of this game with Christina, a 14-year-old with problems related to both anxiety and depression.

THERAPIST: My turn. Let me see. *(Draws card.)* Okay, the situation is this: I am 15 and in 10th grade. My locker is next to a boy whom I like, but I don't really know him yet. He is walking up to his locker and I am feeling really nervous. Whoa—tough one. Let's think this through. Would I want to hide my feelings here?

CHRISTINA: Oh yeah, for sure. Though that's kinda hard to do. I mean, kids notice when another kid is nervous.

THERAPIST: Yeah, it might be tough to hide that feeling. Why would I want to hide my nervousness?

CHRISTINA: I don't know. I mean, if you like the guy, you don't want him to think you're weird by being nervous.

THERAPIST: Okay, so being nervous is weird?

CHRISTINA: Yeah.

THERAPIST: Why is being nervous weird?

CHRISTINA: I don't know. 'Cause being nervous makes you say dumb things . . . you get all shaky.

THERAPIST: Okay, if I was really nervous and I showed that feeling, it could be embarrassing—like if I was shaking all over and saying dumb things. What about if I felt nervous but didn't shake or say dumb things? Would it be okay to be nervous?

CHRISTINA: I guess. I mean, it would be better if you weren't nervous.

THERAPIST: Definitely. I would love to get rid of my nervousness sometimes. How many kids get nervous when they meet someone new that they like?

CHRISTINA: I don't know. Some do, I guess.

THERAPIST: Yeah, I think so. Some do, and maybe even a lot of them do. But let's get back to why would I want to hide my nervous feelings when that guy is coming up to my locker. Sounds like the main reasons are that I could look or say something embarrassing.

CHRISTINA: Right. And it's not cool to be nervous.

THERAPIST: Not to cool to *be* nervous or *show* that I am nervous?

CHRISTINA: Show, I guess, but maybe both?

THERAPIST: Sounds like showing it would have some downsides. But remember what we said about feelings? How they are not like changing the channel on a TV but more like . . . ?

CHRISTINA: Making changes in my room, like cleaning it up a little at a time. Yeah, I remember that.

THERAPIST: Yeah, we can't change how we feel instantly like we can change the TV channels. But if we start taking small steps and keep at it, change usually comes. Okay, time to practice this situation. I will be the girl who is nervous around the boy, and you play the boy, okay?

CHRISTINA: Weird. Um, okay.

THERAPIST: I am going to try it two different ways: once when I show how I am feeling and once when I try not to show it. You try to guess which was which and then we can talk about others way to hide those feelings.

Feelings and Triggers

Trigger	Feeling(s)
Example: Bad grade on test	Sadness, worry, anger
New dog at home	Excitement, happiness
1.	
2.	
3.	
4.	
5.	
6.	
7.	
8.	
9.	
10.	
11.	
12.	

MODULE 3

Empathy Skills

Empathy represents an important aspect of emotional competence because of its role in interpersonal relationships. Developmentally, it is a more mature skill than those described in the previous two modules.

Carolyn Saarni (1999) has written the seminal book on the development of emotional competence. In that book, she describes the importance of empathy in emotional development. For example, she notes that empathic involvement may be one of the most important ingredients for fostering strong relationships. Furthermore, empathy is also a prime driver for many prosocial behaviors. As such, helping children develop empathy is critical. Developmental researchers have identified four different component skills in empathy (see Saarni, 1999, for review), and those four are the focus of this module.

First, though, a few words are needed to distinguish empathy from sympathy and these two from personal distress, as all three are related and represent different combinations of the skills covered in the module. *Personal distress*, the experience of distress when others are distressed, results from a failure to separate oneself from the other's feeling (i.e., the other person's distress becomes one's own). *Sympathy* has been defined as *feeling for* another person. Here, a child recognizes how another person is feeling and can separate herself from that feeling, although there is a lack of a deeper appreciation and understanding of the feeling. Sympathy has a detached quality to it, and so in that way is quite unlike personal distress, where there is an overly attached quality. Sympathy can promote prosocial behavior, but that behavior can feel impersonal. *Empathy* has been defined as *feeling with* another person.

An empathic person knows how another feels and has felt it with that person, but can also separate from the feeling to respond in a helpful way.

WHEN TO USE THIS MODULE

This module is designed for use with clients for whom empathy difficulties are related to their problems. As described in Chapter 2, the development of empathy involves an integration of several strands of emotion knowledge and experience. Thus difficulty with empathy can come in a variety of forms. Some clients will struggle with understanding the perspective of others and thus struggle with knowing the emotion another might be experiencing. Others can understand another's feelings but are so distressed about those feelings they are not able to respond adaptively. Still another group of children are able to sense another's feelings without becoming overly distressed themselves, but are not sure how to respond. The teaching and practice points in this module offer some ways to help bolster empathy skills across this range of difficulties.

OBJECTIVES

Objectives for this module are to teach and practice four different skills related to the development of empathy: (1) recognizing others' feelings by using emotion cues, (2) understanding others' feelings (walking in their shoes), (3) feeling others' feelings (sharing the emotion), and (4) separating from others' feelings in order to help.

Note that the second and third objectives are combined in Step 2 of this module so that there are only three steps described here:

1. Recognize emotions in others.
2. Appreciate and share others' feelings.
3. Separate from others' emotions in order to help.

PROCEDURES

Step 1. Recognizing Emotions in Others

Overview

The first step in the development of empathy is an extension of the skills covered in Module 1 (Emotion Awareness) related to understanding the cues for emotions. Here, the therapist will focus on helping the client develop skills in identifying external and possible internal cues for how *another person* is feeling. In the earlier module, a similar skill was developed, but with more of an emphasis on recognizing the client's own feelings.

Teach

Recognizing Others' Feelings

The teaching points here differ from those in Module 1 in that the goal is to increase awareness of signs for feelings *in others*. This skill also draws on content from Module 2 (Emotion Understanding), especially the skills of knowing the various causes of feelings and understanding that feelings may be hidden. Thus, if a therapist has already covered these modules, work on Step 1 of this module is simplified. If neither Module 1 nor 2 has been covered, then teaching this first step of the Empathy module can be divided into two substeps: external cues of others' emotions and situational cues of others' emotions.

External Cues. These are the facial and bodily signs of another person, indicating that some emotion is being experienced. An easy way to check comprehension of this important skill is to generate a list of emotions and then identify the body signals for each one. Then go back through the list of body signals and ask the client to divide them into three groups: (1) "I could see that one," (2) "I might be able to see that one if I look close," or (3) "I could not notice that one, so I would have to ask the person." Examples for (1) would be a smile or laugh, for (2) would be trembling hands, and for (3) would be butterflies in the stomach. The main idea here is for the client to understand that when others experience feelings, some of the signs are apparent to those watching, others require some detective work, and others may be impossible to detect without asking the person directly.

Situational Cues. In the absence of external cues and in cases in which one is not able to ask a person directly about his or her feelings, understanding how a situation may affect the person can help guide us. In some situations, like talking on the phone or texting back and forth, situational cues become even more important because the body cues are largely or entirely unavailable.

One important aspect of the skill to keep in mind is that people each have idiosyncrasies such that there is not a one-to-one correspondence between situations and feelings. That is, just because one knows the situation does not mean one can know how another person feels in it. There may be any number of character traits, memories or associations, or personal preferences that make one person feel different from another, given the same set of circumstances. In developmental studies that aim to assess how well children can gauge others' feelings, a typical scenario is used: *Tabitha's mother offers to take her bike riding.* The children in the study are asked, "How do you think Tabitha feels about that?" Younger children respond that Tabitha feels happy or excited, because most children enjoy bike riding. However, if the children then learn that Tabitha was afraid of bike riding because she had fallen off her bike once when learning to ride, that information would change how older children predicted her feelings. Younger children, by contrast, sometimes still maintain she will be happy or excited because bike riding is, in their minds, objectively fun.

Practice: Activities and Games

These two games are fun ways to practice identifying emotions using both external and situational clues.

Feelings Jeopardy

Preparation. In advance of the session, the therapist will need to identify at least 11 different video snippets from YouTube or different movies or TV shows the therapist has on DVD or in some other format. (A modified, low-tech version is also possible and is discussed below.) Five of the videos should feature a person physically expressing an emotion. Ideally, at least three different emotions will be expressed at different intensity levels across the five videos. These are called the **Body Signs** videos. Another five videos should feature characters in situations that clearly evoke specific emotions but that do not show the characters making obvious outward signs of their emotions. As with the Body Signs videos, these (the **Situation Signs** videos) will ideally feature a variety of emotions. The 11th video, **Final Jeopardy,** can fit either category but should be the most difficult to guess.

Gameplay. The therapist pretends to be a game-show host, and the client is the contestant. The client is offered a choice of Situation Sign or Body Sign and then shown a random video from the category he choses. The client then guesses the emotion in the scene and is asked to describe *why* he guessed that emotion. The therapist should probe the reasons for maximal teaching value. That is, if the client relies on a single, obvious clue, the therapist should review other more subtle signals. This probing often involves rewatching the video. The idea here is to make each video into a teaching tool.

The game is played in a manner similar to *Jeopardy* such that the videos are associated with point totals and a client can call out, "I'll take Situation Signs for 200." For each correct answer, the client earns points. Correct answers are those that are well justified, as judged by the therapist. The videos chosen may have more than one correct answer. For each incorrect answer, the client loses that number of points. Play continues until all 10 Body Signs and Situation Signs videos have been reviewed. Then the client moves into Final Jeopardy, which is worth 1,000 points.

Feelings Jeopardy can be adapted so that a therapist does not need access to videos. Role playing stories can be used, as well as picture books for younger clients. An important element related to the success of the game is the therapist's advance preparation. Selecting good situations relevant to the client will maximize the utility and value of the game.

Triple Deck Feelings Detective Game

Preparation. Here, the therapist creates three decks of cards. The first deck contains **body signs** for different feelings, the second deck contains **situation signs** for different feelings, and the third deck contains **individual information** for different feelings. The cards may include words alone or can include pictures to help clarify the words on the cards. A deck should contain at least 5 cards in each category; 10 cards per category makes for long and fun playing. Examples for each category of card are provided here.

Body signs

- The person has a funny feeling in her stomach.
- The person has a look of intense concentration on his face.
- The person has his/her hands covering her face and is peeking out between the fingers.

Situation signs

- The boy has just scored a goal in soccer.
- The girl is at the animal hospital with a sick pet.
- The boy is at a school dance and about to ask someone to dance.

Individual information

- She is not at all shy; she is very outgoing and likes to talk in front of groups.
- He is not a very good athlete and does not like to play sports.
- She has had a very bad day.

Gameplay. The three decks are shuffled and stacked separately. Therapist and client take turns alternating between Player and Judge. A turn is played as follows: the Player draws one card from each deck, leaving the cards face down. The Player then chooses how many cards to turn over: one, two, or all three cards. After turning over the card(s), the Player makes a guess about the feeling the person might have and explains why that feeling makes sense. After making the initial guess, all three cards are turned over and the Judge and Player work together to determine whether the Player's guess was correct.

Points are awarded as follows: 50 points for a correct guess with one card; 25 points for a correct guess with two cards; 10 points for a correct guess with all three cards. The first player to reach 200 points wins.

Step 2. Appreciating and Sharing Others' Feelings

Overview

Step 2 combines two similar but separate learning points related to developing empathy: being able to recognize how someone else will feel in a particular situation and being able to "feel" the feeling of the other, to understand more deeply that person's feelings.

Teach

Feeling with Others

The step from *recognizing* another's feelings to *feeling* the other's feelings is paradoxically both small and huge. The same information is needed for both: what the situation is, what the person expresses, and what one knows about the person. Hence, a small step—hardly a new cognitive task. But it is one thing to recognize intellectually the emotion of another and quite another to feel that feeling in a manner similar to how the other person might experience it.

One useful metaphor is to compare a person and a computer. Many clients can explain that a computer can learn to guess emotions in others if the computer is given enough information. Many clients will also appreciate the point that a computer cannot tell what the emotion feels like or how intensely the person might be feeling it. Thus the goal is to help clients learn how to experience another's feelings to the extent that they can appreciate the other person's level of emotion. Another more common metaphor is to help a client learn to walk, almost literally, in another's shoes.

Practice: Activities and Games

Both of the following games are good ways to help clients understand the teaching points related to feeling "with" another.

Emotional Idol

The game here is inspired by a popular television program, *American Idol*, in which contestants engage in singing auditions in front of a panel of judges. In this game, the singing is replaced with acting out emotional scenes. Low-tech and high-tech versions are possible.

Preparation (Low-Tech Version). The therapist develops a set of cards describing scenarios. The deck of cards may grow as the therapist learns and adapts the game to his/her clients' needs and strengths. In the beginning, though, a set of about 10 cards is needed. Each card describes a situation involving a person having an emotional experience. The description should contain enough information to help the player somewhat accurately gauge the emotion of the other person *and* appreciate what the emotional meaning of the situation would be for that specific person. As a result, the following information should be included for each situation described on a card.

- **Identity.** Who is the target person? The person's name, age, gender, and family details (e.g., how many in the family, who is parenting the target) should be provided.
- **Personal information.** In addition to basic demographics about the person, the scenario should also provide some background and personal information (i.e., likes/dislikes, temperament) to help the player understand and appreciate what the person might be like so that person's emotional reaction can be gauged.
- **Situation.** A description of what is happening to the person is needed, with enough details so a client can guess the emotions being experienced.

Another consideration when building the scenarios is to vary the following parameters to permit good and diverse practice of the skill:

- **Emotion.** That is, make sure the cards cover a variety of emotional ground, including, at the very least: anger, sadness, anxiety, and happiness.
- **Intensity.** Similarly, the cards should run the gamut of emotional intensity from weakly felt emotion to intensely experienced feelings.
- **Character demographics.** Vary gender, age (including adults and children), and other relevant variables to help the client understand and appreciate the feelings of a wide variety of others.
- **Proximity.** The cards should also include some feelings and situations that are quite similar to the client's own situation, while others may have less direct relevance.

Included here are four sample scenarios.

Scenario 1: Angela is a 15-year-old who lives with her mother and her two younger brothers. Her dad died when she was 7 years old. Her mother has not remarried, although she has had a few boyfriends. Currently, though, her mother is not dating anyone. A few months ago, the family moved a few miles from their old home and now live in a new town and in a new school district. Angela has always been an outgoing girl who likes to be with her friends. She did not have trouble making new friends at her new school. One day, she is hanging out with friends from her new school at the mall and the friends start complaining about their parents. One friend, Teri, tells the group about how mean her dad is and then asks Angela what her dad is like.

Scenario 2: Tyler is an 11-year-old who lives with his mother and father. He has no brothers or sisters, although his aunt and uncle live nearby with three cousins who are near his age. Tyler has trouble with academics in school, but he excels in art class. Small for his age, he is not a very good athlete. However, he has a good sense of humor and has a number of close friends, most of them kids he has known since preschool. One day, on the playground after school, his friends invite him to join the kickball game. He joins but does not play well, being tagged out after each time he kicks and dropping a few balls while fielding. As the game winds down, it is Tyler's turn to kick. There are two runners on base and his team is down by one run.

Scenario 3: Jessica is a 13-year-old who lives with her mother, father, an older sister who is 17, and a younger brother who is 8. Her parents are both teachers at the local elementary school. Unlike most of the girls in her class, Jessica has not really started puberty yet and has not expressed any interest in boys. She has a few close friends, but many of her classmates consider her a little weird, maybe because she is aloof. One day, Jessica is in the lunchroom, eating by herself because her best friend, Erin, is out sick, when a few female peers walk by, talking loudly. One of them points at Jessica and then the group hides their faces with their hands, laughing.

Scenario 4: José is a 9-year-old who lives with his mother, father, and three older sisters, who are 17, 14, and 12. His father works two jobs and his mother is employed part-time. José is an active boy who is good at sports. He also does well in his classes, although he does not like schoolwork much. José gets along decently with his peers, but he is easily offended by kids who joke around. He has sometimes fought with his peers when they tease him. One day, during language arts class, José is reading aloud from a storybook in the classroom. After mispronouncing a few words, a peer named Manny says, "José, maybe you need glasses?" and the classroom erupts in laughter.

Preparation (High-Tech Version). Instead of cards, a therapist can collect video clips of children, teens, and adults in emotional scenarios. As with the card scenarios, clips that allow variety across the parameters listed earlier is important. When using media, it can also pay to know the preferences of your client and use examples that are familiar and enjoyed by the client. As many therapists know, it can be helpful to watch television geared to the age groups one works with so that a therapist's own familiarity with popular shows can lead to salient examples that will help clients connect with the teaching points.

Gameplay. As noted, the game is based on *American Idol*. As such, the players take turns "trying out" for a part in a movie (or TV show) by acting out emotional scenes based on characters and situations that are depicted on the scenario cards or in the video snippets. The other player(s) serve as the audience. Unlike on *American Idol*, in Emotional Idol, there is no judge and no one wins. Although the game is usually played with a therapist and a single client, the game can also include groups of children and/or families.

Whether using the low- or high-tech version, the game has three phases.

- **Phase 1: Brainstorming.** The first "tryout" player is presented with one of the scenario cards (or videos). The player then uses a brief (i.e., 5 minutes or less) brainstorming period to come up with a list of *body feelings*, *thoughts*, and *actions* that the person having that emotion might be experiencing, based on the scenario. The list is designed to help the player identify things to try when acting out the scene in Phase 2. If the client is the player, the therapist is encouraged to help the client generate the list.
- **Phase 2: Tryout.** Once the brainstorming period is over, the player pretends to get on a stage and then acts out a scene, using the scenario and the brainstorming list as inspiration. The player should be encouraged to exhibit and experience the emotion of the character and not the emotion that the player thinks he himself would have or the emotion the way that he himself would experience it.
- **Phase 3: Rehash.** After the tryout, the players discuss how the scene went, with an emphasis on how accurately the player portrayed the feelings of the character in the scenario. Feedback from the therapist should be gentle and full of praise at first and then suggest an *add-on* for a possible second tryout.

High-Tech Option. Using a video camera to record the tryout can enhance this review of the performance and help the therapist isolate specific moments of the tryout for discussion. The therapist should always remember that the goal is not to make the client a better actor, but rather to help the client have the experience of "feeling like" another person.

During Phase 3, the player may be encouraged to repeat the tryout, with the goal being a performance that the player (and therapist) is satisfied he has accomplished depicting the emotional experience of the character described in the scenario.

Take One, Take Two

This game is an emotion-related variant of Jean Piaget's classic *mountain task*. In the Piaget experiments, a child was seated in front of a table with a set of model mountains arranged to created different views depending on where one was sitting.

In some of the experiments, there were dolls seated in other chairs around the table. After observing from one seat, the child was then shown pictures and asked which picture represented what he saw from his perspective and then which pictures represented what the different dolls would have seen from their perspectives. In this game, the same basic principle is applied, except that instead of asking the client to provide a guess about the visual perspective of others, the focus is on the emotional perspective of others.

Preparation. A deck of cards is needed for this game, with two different types of cards: Situation cards and Person cards. Therapists are encouraged to develop a deck of at least 10 Situation cards and at least 15 Person cards. Following are some tips for good Situation and Person cards, along with several examples of each.

Situation Card Examples and Tips. These cards should describe the interaction of two people. Each description should provide enough details to allow the players to do some perspective taking while also leaving considerable room for a variety of different possible feelings for each person in the situation. In other words, a situation that clearly requires one person to be angry is not a good choice. Here are several examples.

Scenario 1: Two people are on a school bus heading back from a field trip during which the students learned about an important historical place and also got to eat ice cream.

Scenario 2: Two people are at a birthday party together, eating cake and talking.

Scenario 3: Two people are playing in a game of baseball or softball together after school. The game is an important one for the school's team and the score is tied late in the game.

Scenario 4: Two friends are walking home from school in the rain. One person has an umbrella and the other forgot his.

Person Card Examples and Tips. These should contain basic information about one of the two people involved in the situation. Age is not necessary, but name and gender should be provided. The card should clearly state how the person is feeling, including, in most cases, how the person feels toward the other person involved in the situation. It also helps to include additional personal information to help the player understand and appreciate what each person's emotional perspective might be in the situation. It is worth making clear that the Person cards are much more detailed than the Situation cards. Here are several examples.

Sandra. Sandra has had a terrible day. She is tired from not getting enough sleep and she forgot her lunch and so had to eat food her friends gave her. She is feeling particularly irritated with Person 2 because Person 2 did not say hi to her when they got to school.

Paul. Paul is very nervous today because his mother has been sick and she was going in for tests to see if something was really wrong with her. However, Paul also got some good news today: he received an A on his big social studies test. And Paul is feeling excited to hang out with Person 2 because he really likes Person 2.

Ritch. Ritch is feeling bored today. Schoolwork has been pretty easy, and he would rather be home playing with his video games or else reading his new book. He thinks the teacher keeps catching him misbehaving, and as a result he feels really frustrated. When he notices Person 2, he remembers that he has some really cool stuff in his desk or backpack, and so Ritch decides to be nice to Person 2 in the hope that he will share the cool stuff.

Vanessa. Last night, Vanessa performed in the final show of a play in which she had a medium-size part. She is very relieved that the show went well. All day, her classmates have been saying she did a good job, and she is feeling pretty good about herself. However, when she sees Person 2, who had the lead in the play and was really great in it, she starts to feel nervous, hoping that she also will say that Vanessa did a good job.

Gameplay. The first player draws a Situation card, reads the card aloud, and places it face up. She then randomly picks one of the Person cards for herself and another for the other player, being careful not to look at either card. Each of the players silently reads their Person card. Players should not show the card to the other player(s).

Take One. The players then act out the scene described on the Situation card, with each player focusing on demonstrating the emotion on their Person card. Pretending like you are making a movie makes this a bit more fun for some clients. As in a movie, Take One will always be a bit awkward; each player will be unaware of the other player's emotion and the client should be instructed not to say what emotions are on her card.

Debrief One. After the scene, each player guesses what the other player was feeling and *why* he or she was feeling that way. Players are permitted to ask each other questions to clarify and/or suggest other emotions, but the players should refrain from sharing what was written on the Person cards.

Take Two. After the first debrief, the players switch Person cards and replay the scene.

Debrief Two. After the second take, the players talk over what it was like to switch roles. Instead of focusing on the identification of emotion, the discussion should focus on the experience of "being" and "feeling like" the other person.

Step 3. Separating from Others' Emotions in Order to Help

Overview

The next and last step in the development of empathy is separating oneself from feeling with the others so as to be able to help. The overall teaching message is twofold: it can help to be a better friend if one is able to feel with the friend, and because one wants to help the friend who might be having a tough time, one cannot feel too strongly with him or her. When the goal is empathy, one must tread into the *dangerous* territory of "feeling with" in order to most appropriately offer empathic assistance.

Teach

Separation Can Help You Help Others

As empathy develops, there develops also an appreciation for the nuance of helping someone in an emotional situation. Indeed, one of the important lessons of the module is that everyone sees and experiences situations from a different perspective. The emotional world is not a one-size-fits-all arrangement. Along those lines, teaching clients how to help their friends when their friends are feeling emotional involves making it clear that helping others involves a *fitting* process, wherein one attempts to determine what will work best for a particular person. Thus, throughout the development of empathy, there is an emphasis on perspective taking.

A related point to emphasize here is how someone else's emotions can make one emotional. Awareness of the fact that one can get emotional when others are emotional helps in being able to complete the separation enough so that one can respond empathically but effectively. As the astute reader can guess, this teaching point leads naturally into the modules on emotion regulation that follow (i.e., Modules 4 through 8). For clients whose emotion regulation skills are relatively strong, empathic responding comes more easily. However, for some clients this last step in empathy may come with difficulty. In fact, for clients with limited emotion regulation skills, it may be best to cover the emotion regulation modules before the empathy module.

The Pros and Cons of Empathy

Another teaching point concerns the pros and cons of empathy. That is, *feeling with* someone can have emotional consequences for the person empathizing. It can be productive to conduct an unbiased and Socratic analysis of being empathic with clients, helping them sort through the benefits and downsides of empathy. For most clients, the analysis can be conducted at a broad level: "What are some good things and some bad things about being empathic?" This broad perspective is useful for most clients whose potential empathic "recipients" function relatively well. In such cases, the general point here would be that empathy generally has more benefits than costs, although there may be exceptions. On occasion, though, it can help to conduct this cost–benefit analysis in a more granular way, considering the impact of experiencing empathy for different people in the client's life. Specifically, for some clients there may be particular people with whom empathy *costs more* than it does with others.

As one example, feeling with a particularly distressed and disturbed peer or family member may be more taxing and beyond the client's skill set. In such cases, the therapist may praise the client for efforts to empathize with the distressed individual but note that sometimes professional help may be warranted.

Practice: Activities and Games

This game allows clients to practice separating from another person rather than "feeling with" that person in order to help.

Call-In Radio Show

The game is designed to resemble a call-in radio show. The game requires two players, with one person playing the role of the caller and the other playing the role of the host.

Preparation. The therapist will need scenarios written on cards to use as part of the call-in show. Each card needs the following information:

- **Situation.** A situation must be described in adequate detail to help the caller set the scene and also provide enough clues so the host might reasonably guess the emotion.
- **Personal information.** The cards should also provide the caller with information about the character, including demographics as well as relevant historical information. These data must be sufficient to help the caller get into character as well as provide some guidance to the host for guessing the emotion as well as offering help.
- **Emotion.** The card should also explicitly state the caller's emotion. Although

the caller will not reveal this during the call, it is important for the caller to understand clearly what emotion she should convey.

Several examples of the scenario cards follow.

Scenario 1: You are Dolores, a 13-year-old who is very upset because your best friend, Kamilla, is moving away in a week. You are a shy person and have trouble making friends, so you are not sure how you are going to ever have a friend like Kamilla again.

Scenario 2: You are Toby, a 14-year-old whose mother and father are getting divorced. Although you are glad that they might stop fighting all the time, you worry that you won't get to see your dad very much because he is threatening to move out of the state. You are also mad at your parents in general because when they are not fighting, they are bugging you about how you don't do your chores and are not getting good enough grades.

Scenario 3: You are Carmela, a 16-year-old whose boyfriend has not called you back since last night and you are worried that he might be losing interest in you. He usually calls or texts you back right away. Also, because you lost your driving privileges for being late on curfew last weekend, you cannot drive to his house. He lives too far away for you to bike or walk there.

Scenario 4: You are Kyle, an 11-year-old whose best friend, Hanley, is always getting picked on by the other boys in your class. You don't know how to help Hanley, and you are also worried that the other kids are going to start teasing and bullying you more.

Gameplay. Cards are shuffled and then fanned out face down on a flat surface. Players take turns as caller and host. The caller selects a scenario card from the deck, keeping it hidden, and then pretends to call in to the show. The host answers the call, and the caller then describes the scenario in his own words. However, the caller must *not* reveal his emotions, instead focusing on revealing personal information and information about the situation. The caller can add information to the situation that is not on the card. The host has the tough job, with her goal being to complete the following tasks:

- **Show empathy.** The host should guess the caller's emotion or emotions, providing a detailed description as to how she arrived at the guess. The goal is for the host to stay in character while doing this; however, for some clients this is too difficult at first. In such cases, the therapist can call *time-out* and have a "meeting" where the client and therapist think through the situation together and identify the emotional options.

- **Offer help.** The next step is for the host to offer some help in the form of practical advice or verbal support. Again, some clients are able to do this in character whereas others benefit from a *time-out,* during which they discuss ways to accomplish this goal.

For clients who like to play for points, after the call is complete the caller can give the host up to 5 points for the empathy and help efforts; that is, up to 10 points per call. Therapists should remember that shaping is a key goal and thus praise and reward early efforts despite imperfections, with a longer-term goal being to shape the direction and quality of the client's responses. Gameplay can continue until one player reaches a particular score (e.g., 20).

MODULE 4

Emotion Regulation Skills I
Prevention Skills

The remaining five modules are devoted to emotion regulation, in large part due to the construct's complexity and the variety of strategies that can be used to teach it. The first two emotion regulation modules (this one and the next) present strategies that could be referred to as *antecedent management*; they offer emotion regulation skills to designed to prevent future problems. The final three modules focus on regulation processes that can be used during or after a stressor or challenge and are aimed, primarily, at helping clients regulate "in the moment."

The modules on emotion regulation come after those on emotion awareness, emotion understanding, and empathy because, in theory, regulation comes *after* these emotional development achievements. Of course, as noted in Chapter 2, that is oversimplifying emotional development. For these five modules, the emphasis is on what Kopp (1989) referred to as the "planful regulation" of emotion.

The first two modules might be summarized by the adage "an ounce of prevention is worth a pound of cure." They adapt strategies from a variety of sources, leaning particularly on Linehan's treatment for clients with borderline personality disorder (Linehan, 1993) and her focus on two broad categories of "prevention" skills: "Your body as a temple" and "Doing things you are good at."

Viewing one's body as a temple will be a familiar idea to those who recall Abraham Maslow's hierarchy of needs. Maslow posited that human "needs" were arranged in a hierarchical fashion such that one could only yearn for "higher" needs if "lower" needs were met. For Maslow, the "lowest" level needs were called *physiological needs*. Here, he included our need for food, water, sleep, and shelter, among other biologically driven base needs. The second-level needs he called *safety needs* and included safety of the self and family as well as ready access to resources, through employment, for example. Next were the *love/belonging needs*, including

155

friendship and family connections. The fourth-level needs, the *esteem needs*, represent our needs for self-confidence, self-esteem, and achievement as well respect for and of others. Finally, Maslow posited a fifth level, called *self-actualization*. Here, a person yearns for a moral, creative, and spontaneous life.

Although Maslow's theory has its detractors, it is nevertheless instructive when observing child behavior (and adult behavior, including one's own) to consider the status of the lower needs. This is particularly true when considering emotion regulation. For many (all?), lack of food, sleep, or a lack of stability in our lives can increase the sensitivity of our emotional "alarms." People are more easily set off in situations that would not generally "get to" them when their basic needs are not well met.

Those readers who have parented or spent long days with children have likely had the experience of seeing a child "melt down." It could be at the mall or on an outing, often an enjoyable one. At first, during the meltdown, an adult may try to reason with the child and search his or her own mind for the logical explanation for the upset. Even when the adult seems to have found the "right" answer (e.g., provides a desired stuffed animal that has fallen), the upset does not abate. It may be that the adult then realizes, "Oh—you are hungry (or tired or stressed by a specific change)." Although attending to the "lower" need(s) will not immediately end the upset, doing so does begin to right the ship. And often being mindful of and attending to those lower needs can be a great first defense against extreme emotional upset. Accordingly, this module is designed to orient clients and their caregivers to the importance of taking care of the physical self as a way to deal with feelings.

WHEN TO USE THIS MODULE

This module is designed for use when a therapist believes a major contributor to a client's emotion regulation difficulties is one or more of the following: (1) poor sleep habits, (2) poor eating habits, (3) lack of exercise, or (4) poor health-maintenance skills.

OBJECTIVES

The objectives for this module are to teach and practice four different skills that are designed to improve physical functioning and health, thereby making the client less prone to emotion dysregulation:

1. Eating well and healthily.
2. Engaging in exercise and activities.
3. Developing good sleep hygiene.
4. Maintaining physical health.

PROCEDURES

The following module contains five steps. Step 1 may be worth considering for use with every client, but therapists are encouraged to use assessment data to guide selection of appropriate interventions. Steps 2 through 5 should be used only when they are relevant for the client.

Step 1. Regulating Emotion: An Introduction

Overview

The first step is designed to address and justify why emotion regulation is a relevant topic for therapy.

Teach

Dealing with Feelings Requires Flexibility and Persistence

There Are Many Strategies—and No "Right" One. This point can be divided into two subpoints: (1) there are many ways to deal with feelings, and (2) there is no surefire right strategy that will work every time. If this is the first module in the book being used with a client, a few quick activities may be helpful (see the next Practice section). For clients already exposed to earlier modules, though, this teaching point can often be made didactically and/or Socratically.

. . . And Sometimes, More Than One Strategy Is Needed. Because there is no universal solution for dealing with emotions, often multiple efforts and multiple strategies are needed. There are myriad metaphors to convey this point. For example, in video games the character often faces challenges. As the levels become more difficult, the number of different strategies needed to "win" the level increases. The therapist can also convey that sometimes multiple strategies must be used in sequence to achieve success. That is, one may need to follow a set of steps (often in a precise sequence), akin to following a recipe to bake cookies in which the step of putting the cookies in the oven should come after making the dough. In that same way, some situations generate distressing feelings that will ultimately require a set of sequential strategies, rather than one single strategy, in order to regain emotional stability.

Practice: Activities and Games

Emotion-Coping Story Building

Here, the client and therapist work together to create a story that involves a child encountering a set of emotionally taxing situations.

Preparation. The therapist should have on hand a set of index cards or sheets of paper on which to record the emotionally taxing situations, or the therapist may wish to prepare these situations ahead of time. The situations do not need to be complex but should reflect a diversity of emotions as well as a variety of emotion intensities. Also, it can be wise to include some situations relevant to the client's own life, as well as other situations that are not relevant. The storytelling can be done verbally, in written form, using pictures (e.g., comic strip) or other art forms (e.g., diorama), or using puppets or other figures. The stories can be recorded (audio or video) to review later with the client or parents. Thus, depending on the medium used to play the game, the therapist might need art supplies, puppets or other props, or even a video- or audio-recording device on hand.

Examples of emotional situations are listed here. The same character name is used throughout because the goal is to create a story about one child.

Scenario 1: Pat has just received a very bad grade on an important exam.

Scenario 2: Pat's sibling just took and broke (by accident) an important item from Pat's room.

Scenario 3: Pat's best friend has just moved to another state.

Scenario 4: Pat's parents have been arguing a lot lately.

Scenario 5: Pat saw that her steady boyfriend just accepted a Facebook friend request from a someone who has a crush on him.

Gameplay. There are two basic ways to play the game. The first is straightforward and easy to use with most clients. Here, the therapist and client select one of the situations and then build a story together. The therapist's primary role is to ensure that the story highlights the two teaching points of this step: that there are many ways to deal with feelings, and that sometimes the first thing one tries does not work—persistence is often needed. A good way to accomplish this goal is for the therapist to suggest that the client consider an alternative ending to the story, one in which a different "dealing with feelings" path was undertaken. As noted above, the story can be generated in any medium that best fits the client.

Alternate Version: Taking Turns. A variation of the game may be useful for clients who find a large project like building a story to be daunting. This variation is also good for clients who struggle with the first version either because of limited coping ideas or else a tendency to be overly goofy or oppositional. In this variation, the therapist and client take turns building the story sentence by sentence (or picture by picture). Here the unfolding of the narrative is a mystery, and the story-building method permits a lot of opportunity for the therapist to offer corrective feedback throughout. Again, the therapist's role is to guide the process toward making the two primary teaching points of this Step 1. The case example of 11-year-old Ellie illustrates this "taking turns" way to play the game.

THERAPIST: Okay, we are going to write a story together about a kid who copes with a tough situation by dealing with her feelings. I have some cards here with situations. Will you pick one card, please?

ELLIE: Okay. *(Draws a card.)*

THERAPIST: *(reading)* Pat has just received a very bad grade on an important exam. Tough one.

ELLIE: What do we do?

THERAPIST: Well, we pretend like we are writers, like for a book or a TV show. And we are going to tell the story of what happens to Pat. I'll get us started. Let's pretend like we are writing this for a TV show. What channel will our show be on?

ELLIE: Maybe Nick or Disney Channel, since it's about a kid?

THERAPIST: Great—let's do Nickelodeon. Okay, I am going to tell one part of the story, and then you can tell what you think happens next. And we'll take turns until we see how Pat deals with her feelings about this test. I will write our story down here. Okay, so here I go. *(writing and talking out loud)* "Pat is sitting at her desk looking at her test with the ugly grade of a D on it. She is feeling very sad and mad, too." Now it's your turn. Just tell me a sentence or two about what happens next.

ELLIE: Um. Hmm. Well, she gets up and goes to the school bus.

THERAPIST: Great! Okay. I wonder what she does on the bus? Does she talk to anyone? Or tell anyone about the D?

ELLIE: No. She just sits by herself and doesn't talk to anyone.

THERAPIST: *(writing)* Fantastic. So the bus pulls up to Pat's stop and she gets off and trudges home.

Step 2. Eating—and Eating Healthy

Overview

The point here is not to convince clients to eat better. Instead, the therapist discusses with the client and his parents, ideally in Socratic fashion, how and why healthful eating helps regulate emotion. In general, the most reasonable aim is for small changes in diet rather than a complete restructuring of the client's eating habits. For example, if a client adds one more vegetable or fruit per day to his diet, the therapist should praise the small change rather than bemoan the fact that the recommendation is for five such servings daily.

Teach

Why Eating Healthfully Matters for Feelings

Eating healthfully and regularly promotes physiological well-being. If one's body is in balance, it is easier (although not necessarily easy) to handle stressors. On a personal note, several colleagues and I like to refer to being "*hangry*" (i.e., hungry plus angry) when our moods are being negatively affected by our hunger.

Practice: Activities and Games

Online Games

Because of the public health ramifications of childhood obesity, government agencies have developed many tools to promote healthy eating habits in children. Internet-based games can be found at many websites, including the following:

- *www.fns.usda.gov/tn*
- *school.fueluptoplay60.com*
- *www.choosemyplate.gov*

Monitoring

Therapists can suggest that the client and/or parents monitor the client's eating along with some indices of functioning (e.g., mood, activity level, or frequency of getting into trouble). By tracking those data one can test whether there is a link that may be worth addressing. The **Eating Diary (Handout 1)** provides one way to monitor food and mood.

Family Mealtimes

Recent research has demonstrated a "fact" that may seem like common sense to some: families who regularly eat meals together function better and eat more healthily. Thus learning more about the meal habits of clients' families may help to identify ways to improve healthy eating. Family mealtimes not only promote healthy eating, but also offer opportunities for families to communicate and share, thereby creating the chance for improving emotional health. Work by Barbara Fiese and her colleagues (e.g., Fiese, Foley, & Spagnola, 2006) has been particularly instructive in this domain. They have identified some important ingredients to effective family mealtimes: (1) clear, direct, and supportive communication; (2) flexible and smooth transitions before, during, and after mealtimes; (3) openness to sharing of emotions; and (4) empathic involvement in the concerns of family members. Some tips for helping parents and caregivers to plan successful family mealtimes are given below.

FAMILY MEALTIME TIPS

Have healthy foods on hand. Helping a caregiver plan menus and snacks, and even helping them create a shopping list, are good strategies.

Open your table. Inviting the children's friends to join the family table from time to time may improve children's enthusiasm for family mealtimes.

Be a healthy eating role model. Help caregivers think through how they can integrate healthy eating into their own behaviors, particularly during family mealtimes, but also at other times of the day.

Involve children in food preparation. Although not all children enjoy preparing food, many do. Being involved in preparing a meal or snack may make the child more willing to try a new food. For younger children, clear and limited tasks are often best. For example, younger children can obtain ingredients from the pantry and/or measure them. Older children can be involved in more complex tasks such as planning and/or preparing one item in a meal, or perhaps even the entire meal. In addition to helping children learn about healthy eating, involving them in meal preparation is a chance for them to learn an important life skill.

Step 3. Getting Active!

Overview

Aside from the obvious health benefits, exercise can be a terrific technique to include in therapy because many clients are glad for the chance to get out of their classroom or a therapy office to shoot hoops, jump rope, or engage in other physical activities. For this step, obviously, practice takes precedence over lecture-style teaching.

Teach

Being Active Helps One Deal with Feelings

The first point to make is that exercise is clearly good for the body. Large-scale studies have documented that exercise has important physical health benefits. The second but less obvious point is that there are mental health benefits to exercise as well (Callaghan, 2004; Fox, 1999; Stathopoulou, Powers, Berry, Smits, & Otto, 2006). In studies of adults, exercise as a stand-alone intervention yielded strong benefits, particularly for depressed clients (Fox, 1999; Stathopoulou et al., 2006). Evidence also supports the idea that exercise has both physical and mental health benefits for

children, although there are fewer studies (e.g., Ortega et al., 2008). The idea here is
to convey to the client (and parents, if appropriate) that exercise may help one deal
with feelings in a few ways:

- It may help people burn off steam or decompress after a long day.
- It may help people feel good about themselves because they have taken care
  of themselves.
- It may help people feel more relaxed and thus better able to handle stressors.

Practice: Activities and Games

Here is one way to help the client think through various exercise options and follow
through with the one most likely to be feasible and fun.

Make a List and Schedule the Activity

Before a therapist can suggest and plan for an increased activity level for the client,
the therapist and client need to establish some goals for increased activity/exercise.
And those goals are not possible without a list of activities that are potentially
attractive to the client and also feasible for the family. Thus this activity involves
generating a list of activities that the client *could* try. The therapist can portray
the list as a menu. Because some children excel in team-oriented activities (like
baseball or basketball), whereas others do better with individually driven activities (like running or tennis), any list should include both team sport and individual
options. Ratings can help winnow the initial list to a smaller group of possible
activities.

A good rule of thumb is to build a list that includes several activities, with at
least one activity meeting *each* of the following criteria:

- Free or very low cost
- Already familiar to the client
- Of interest to the client
- Accessible year-round (i.e., not snow skiing for those living in temperate cli-
  mates)
- Possible to do daily
- 15–20 minutes in duration
- Possible to practice with the client during session time

For times when a therapist is challenged in making the list, there are good
websites that provide lists of activities. For example, the Centers for Disease Control and Prevention website has a quiz to help guide activity selection. The site also
includes a customizable activity calendar. The President's Council on Physical Fitness also has an online list.

Once the list is built, the therapist will work with the client to identify the activities that represent the best candidates for immediate scheduling. It is important to help temper the overzealous client (or caregiver) who wants to schedule an activity every day. In general, it is best to scale back ambition in favor of having immediate and slow success. Similarly, encourage the languorous client who wants to choose nothing to give one activity a try—even if that effort needs to come during the therapy session. In general, aim low at first, with the hope that the benefits of physical activity become clear. Then, as the success of your experiment mounts, the therapist can suggest that the client add to her repertoire. The **Activity Diary** (**Handout 2**) can help link activity level to mood.

One particularly useful way to conclude this list making is to select one of the activities on the list and try it out during the meeting time, with ratings before and after the attempt to see what effect it had on the client's mood (or energy level or other relevant marker). As with the advice just given, set expectations low. For example, if the activity is soccer, the therapist and client could kick a soccer ball back and forth in a hallway for a few minutes.

In the following case example, a therapist generates a list of possible activities with an 11-year-old client, Marc, and his mother. Marc is a depressed and oppositional boy who is moderately overweight. His favorite activity is playing video games.

THERAPIST: *(to mother)* Sounds like getting more active might be something worth exploring with Marc. *(to Marc)* What are some activities that come to mind that you could do to get more active, Marc?

MARC: Video games! Does that count?

MOTHER: *(Shakes head, starts to speak.)*

THERAPIST: Sure, let's write that one down. Right now we're brainstorming. We won't pick what the best things are to do right now. We'll just list some out.

MARC: Cool! Video games are great!

MOTHER: Soccer.

MARC: I hate soccer.

THERAPIST: Hold on—let me write soccer down. We can wait on "scoring" these until after we get our list. Okay?

MARC: All right, but I hate soccer.

THERAPIST: So what else? *(long silence)* Okay. Coming up with ideas can be tough. Let's play a game with this. I will give some characteristics of an activity and you name something that fits what you like. Ready? *(Marc nods)* Something you can do outside.

MARC: Video games—you can play those outside.

THERAPIST: Right. I have video games. What is something else you can do outside?

MARC: Bike riding.

THERAPIST: Okay, bike riding. More outside things?

MOTHER: Football?

THERAPIST: That is another outside one. We're cooking now!

MARC: Fishing?

THERAPIST: Bingo. Hey, what are some of your favorite video games, Marc?

MARC: I like the Batman game. *Uncharted* is awesome. *Portal.*

THERAPIST: Cool. So, in *Uncharted*, what are you doing?

MARC: The guy in the game is an explorer, and he's solving puzzles, running around shooting people to find a map and get some treasures.

THERAPIST: Cool. Sounds like there are some activities in there you could do in real life. Like running around—that could be playing tag or capture the flag, right?

MARC: Yeah, I guess.

THERAPIST: And using a map to find hidden treasure is a lot like something called geocaching. Have you heard of that?

MARC: No.

THERAPIST: Well, it's like a treasure hunt. There are clues hidden around and you have to find them using tools like a GPS or a compass. If we end up picking it, we can talk more about it.
    Okay, let's shift gears. How about something you can do when the weather is bad?

MARC: Watch TV.

THERAPIST: Got it—watch TV. What's another one?

MOTHER: We have trouble with that—when the weather is cold or rainy. Lots of TV and video games.

THERAPIST: Hmm, let's see what we can come up with. *(long silence)* I make these sorts of lists a lot so I can think of a few. How about swimming in an indoor pool? How about going to the school gym to play basketball? Or running on an indoor track? Or you could bundle up for an outdoor walk?

MARC: Swimming is cool. Could we do that one?

MOTHER: You know, grandpa used to do sit-ups and push-ups inside all winter when I was a kid.

THERAPIST: Yep, that's a great one too—indoor exercising. Okay, we have a good list going. Now, let's go through it and each of you give me two different ratings for each one. First, tell me how much you like the activity and want to do it—or for you, Ms. X, how much you want Marc to do it. Then tell me how easy or hard it would be for your family to coordinate the activity. We can use a 0 to 10 scale for each one. Zero means you hate it, or it would be really hard. Ten would be you love it or else it would be really easy to do it. Make sense? Okay, video games were first.

Step 4. Sleeping Well

Overview

Problems with sleep hygiene are common across the lifespan, and there is growing interest in the interplay of sleep and psychopathological conditions (e.g., Chorney, Detweiler, Morris, & Kuhn, 2008; Harvey, Mullin, & Hinshaw, 2006). Sleep as a specific component of treatment for psychopathology is rarely found in the scientific literature for children and adolescents; however, a reasonable amount of research has been done to test the effects of interventions that target sleep behaviors for children who present with specific sleep-related problems (Mindell, Owens, & Carskadon, 1999). Most of these interventions target the reduction of parental reinforcement of child non-sleep behaviors through extinction procedures. In other words, some studies have suggested that when a child has trouble sleeping at night and is frequently calling his or her parents into the room and/or co-sleeping, an effective intervention involves convincing the parents to ignore the child (except in cases of injury or illness) during specified nighttime hours in order to eliminate the "non-sleep" behavior. Two other common interventions include parental education (particularly preventively), and establishing and rewarding bedtime routines.

Teach

Good Sleep Hygiene Makes It Easier to Deal with Feelings

This step is primarily educational, and the teaching points are probably best discussed with the parents or caregivers rather than the child, as this step does not lend itself well to the Activities and Games theme of most of the modules.

Establish a Bedtime Routine. Many readers will be familiar with families who do not enforce a regular bedtime, even on school nights. Some children appear to function adequately when given the freedom to go to bed whenever they wish, but others are less able to regulate themselves when given free choice on bedtime. In addition, many children need "wind-down" time before bed or thrive best with the structure of a bedtime routine. It can be worth pointing out to parents that predictability and controllability are two important characteristics of effective anxiety reduction strategies.

To understand a family's bedtime routine and zero in on how to improve it, the therapist may want to get a longer view of the evening timeline, including homework schedule, dinnertime, chores, and after-dinner activities. If a therapist perceives that sleep may be related to some of the client's difficulties, the following specific suggested bedtime routine procedures may be helpful.

1. **Make the bedtime clear.** For example, "Bedtime is at 9:00 P.M."
2. **Announce bedtime in advance.** For example, a caregiver can say, "Bedtime is in 15 minutes."
3. **Create a bedtime routine.** This might include:
   - A shower or bath (although some children prefer bathing in the morning).
   - Getting changed into pajamas.
   - Brushing teeth.
   - Engaging in a quiet activity, like storytime or a calm game, one-on-one (if possible) in the child's room.
   - Turning off the lights at the appointed bedtime.
   - Saying a final goodnight or tucking the child into bed can be a good addition.

Make the Bedroom and Bedtime Sleep-Friendly. As much as possible, a bedroom should be a place for sleeping. Access to media in a bedroom is not a necessity and can often harm good sleep hygiene. A few tips to make for a sleep-inducing bedroom and bedtime:

- **Quiet.** Keep the room and nearby rooms quiet. Encourage other family members to use lower voices and keep TV and/or music volumes low. Headphone use is also a good suggestion. Alternatively, white-noise makers can be helpful in some situations and can be purchased inexpensively.
- **Dark.** There is some evidence that sleep quality is better when the bedroom is dark. Encourage the family to create a dark sleeping space for the child. Night lights should be used only if required for safety or as a temporary measure for fearful sleepers working toward darkened sleep.
- **Comfortable.** An obvious suggestion, but it is surprising how uncomfortable some sleeping arrangements can be. Ensure that the child has access to pillows and blankets as needed and that the room is well ventilated.
- **Safe.** Ensure that the child both *is* and *feels* safe in his or her room.

Offer Nonmedical Sleep "Aids." There are numerous nonmedical sleep aids that can be used to help the client who has difficulty initiating or maintaining sleep. These include:

- Sleep-inducing beverages (e.g., warm milk, warm water)
- Back rub
- Hair brushing
- Calming music
- Relaxation exercises (e.g., diaphragmatic breathing)

Promote Physical Activity during the Day. Being active during the day helps a person feel ready to rest. However, it is important to remember (and remind parents) that most children have higher needs for physical activity compared to (most) adults. Encourage caregivers to focus on the needs of their children as separate from their own. Sometimes, caregivers think, "Wow, am I tired? I bet Xavier is tired too." However, the truth may be that Xavier is nowhere near as tired as the caregiver. Vigorous activity during the bedtime routine should generally be avoided, especially for clients who have trouble relaxing. But working with a caregiver to ensure the client has the chance to be physically active during the day can go a long way toward making sleep time more successful. There are also some calm-inducing activities like yoga or stretching that may be appropriate for practicing before bedtime.

Avoid Overstimulating or Emotional Activities before Bed. Like the physical activities just discussed, emotional conversations or situations can make falling asleep more difficult. Furthermore, watching TV, using the computer, and/or playing video games near bedtime can be stimulating and make it difficult for a client to relax. Restricting or forbidding media use around bedtime is often a prudent policy. For some families, this is challenging because the client has unfettered access to media in the form of a bedroom TV or computer. Helping families create and adhere to a media policy for their home is often a helpful step. Collaborate with families to create a policy that is both consonant with the family's values and also enforceable.

Getting Better Sleep (Handout 3) is a useful resource for families working on helping their child learn better sleep habits. The therapist may want to give a copy to caregivers as a reminder of the topics covered in this conversation.

Step 5. Getting Healthy and Staying Healthy

Overview

It is a no-brainer that an illness can interfere with emotional functioning. Nearly every reader can recall being moody or crabby when, for example, sick with a cold or experiencing lower-back pain.

Teach

Staying Healthy Makes It Easier to Deal with Feelings

As with Step 4, the primary points are mostly educational, and the step does not lend itself well to child-centered games and activities. It may be helpful to discuss the following guidelines for maintaining optimal health with caregivers and often with clients, too.

Prevention. The client should have regular contact with a physician to maintain his or her physical health. Sometimes encouraging families to seek regular, preventive medical care for their children requires the therapist to help connect the family to area medical professionals specializing in family medicine and/or pediatrics. A healthy client has one less "stressor" to reduce emotion regulation capacity.

Treatment of Acute Problems. When an acute medical problem emerges, the best advice is to get it treated as soon as possible. Small medical issues can become more complicated when left untreated. Colds and the flu, seasonal afflictions, and generally minor annoyances can allow secondary infections to creep in, causing more serious problems. Not every acute medical problem requires a doctor visit, but ignoring medical problems as they emerge flirts with larger problems later. Most relevant here, a nagging medical problem can reduce a client's capacity for handling stressors. Although therapists cannot and should not provide medical advice, they can provide a client with resources, such as referring families to local medical professionals or suggesting specific written or online materials, to use when making choices about a client's health.

Treatment of Chronic Problems. Chronic medical problems are unfortunately common among children, and there are a few things to keep in mind when working with clients who have them.

Learn and Ask Questions. Just because a doctor is monitoring and treating a child's chronic medical problem does not give the therapist license to remain uninformed about the problem, especially if the problem can affect mental health. Talk with the family about what they know. Be curious and open to learning about the problem from the family—one doesn't need to be the expert on the medical issue. The questions a therapist asks and the interest shown serve several purposes. First, the therapist learns more about the family and their functioning around the illness. Second, the therapist can help the family feel empowered about their level of knowledge. Third, the therapist can assess the family's level of understanding and, if needed, address gaps.

Even with good information from the family, it is a wise policy to maintain consultation with the treating medical provider. Assuming one has the appropriate legal releases, regular contact with the medical provider can even allow a therapist and medical provider to support each other's work. It can also help the family feel supported if there is a team of professionals working to help them to succeed.

Finally, it is worth noting that the therapist should spend time learning about the client's condition from an accurate source. The National Institutes of Health has a website with accurate and updated information about most illnesses: *www.nlm. nih.gov/medlineplus.*

Encourage Adherence. Failure to follow treatment recommendations is a critical problem in medical care. Some chronic problems require regular interventions that are onerous or annoying to children and their families. Avoiding those interventions is often associated with the elimination of unpleasantness: the trap of negative reinforcement has been sprung! Although therapists are not (usually) medical providers, they can inquire about adherence and encourage clients to seek support (from the therapist, from their doctors) when they are having trouble. Therapists can also problem-solve with families around difficulties in adherence. Considerable current research is focused on how behavioral interventions can help individuals with chronic medical conditions manage their illnesses effectively. Sometimes a fresh set of eyes can help the family see a solution to what seemed like an insurmountable challenge that was preventing treatment adherence.

As noted with regard to acute illness, when people don't feel well physically, they don't "do well" mentally and psychologically. Coping capacities are easily taxed and people are more likely to be irritable and impatient. Indeed, some medical problems, when untreated or poorly treated, have direct consequences on one's emotional life, making one angrier or more depressed. In this way, treating medical problems is an important form of emotion regulation.

Eating Diary

Use a mood rating from 0–10, where 0 is the most sad/grumpy mood and 10 is the most happy mood.

Day	Mealtime	Meal	Mood Before	Mood After
Example: Monday 4/10	7:15 PM	Spaghetti and bread	3 (really hungry)	6 (still had homework to do)

Activity Diary

Use a mood rating from 0–10, where 0 is the most sad/grumpy mood and 10 is the most happy mood.

Day	Activity	Time spent	Mood Before	Mood After
Example: Wed. March 2	*Walked dog*	*15 minutes*	*4*	*7*

Getting Better Sleep

1. **Build a Bedtime Routine.**

   Time. Establish a bedtime for each night and stick to it. The amount of sleep a child needs varies depending on the child. Some children are alert and happy with 8 hours a night whereas others need at least 10 hours to be alert the next day. Use what you know about your child to establish the bedtime.

   Transition. Create a bedtime transition time in the family schedule. Focus on relaxing play about 30–60 minutes before bedtime.

   Sleep Preparation Activity. Establish a relaxing bedtime activity, such as giving your child a warm bath or reading him or her a story. Use that same routine daily.

2. **No Big Meals.** Avoid feeding children big meals close to bedtime.

3. **No Caffeine.** Avoid caffeinated drinks and even chocolate too close to bedtime (4–6 hours).

4. **Comfortable Temperature.** Set the bedroom temperature so that it's comfortable—not too warm and not too cold.

5. **Darkness Is Good for Sleep.** Make sure the bedroom is dark. If necessary, use a small night light.

6. **Quiet Hours.** Keep the noise level in the home low once a child is in bed. Encourage older children and other adults to speak softly. Headphones can be useful for music and television in small homes and apartments.

7. **No Naps.** For older children, avoid naps during the day; it can disturb the normal pattern of sleep and wakefulness.

8. **Exercise.** Physical activity during the day promotes good sleep at night.

   Vigorous exercise should be taken in the morning or late afternoon.

   A relaxing exercise can be done before bed to help initiate a restful night's sleep.

9. **Reduce Emotional or Stimulating Situations.** Try to avoid emotionally upsetting conversations and activities before trying to go to sleep. Also, avoid TV or other media that will tend to stimulate and potentially aggravate a child.

MODULE 5

Emotion Regulation Skills II
Mastery

This module shares similarities with the previous one insofar as both are primarily prevention-oriented regulation strategies, or antecedent management. As with Module 4, this module also borrows strategies from a variety of sources, leaning particularly on Linehan's (1993) treatment for clients with borderline personality disorder. In short, the goal of Module 5 is to help clients learn to do things at which they excel.

WHEN TO USE THIS MODULE

This module is designed for use when a therapist hypothesizes that the client either (1) does not have enough activities at which he or she excels or (2) does not spend enough time doing those things at which he or she excels to experience boosts to self-efficacy.

As one example, imagine a client whose primary activity is video games. Although he may excel at video games, the lack of other activities may lead him to feel bored and down when he is not playing. Also, time spent on video games leaves less time for him to engage in other activities from which he can experience mastery.

OBJECTIVES

Objectives for this module are to teach about and practice ways to achieve and sustain a feeling of mastery with an activity.

PROCEDURES

Step 1. Regulating Emotion: An Introduction

If Step 1 from Module 4 has not already been covered with the client, the therapist can use material from it as an introduction to the utility of emotion regulation. If therapists have already covered the material, though, there is no need to repeat it unless the client could benefit from the review.

Step 2. Mastery: Doing Things You Are Good At

Overview

Few will fault the logic of this intervention: most people receive mental health benefits from doing things they are good at. There are two interventions found in treatments for depression that cover similar ground: "activity selection" and "skill building" (e.g., Chorpita & Weisz, 2009). The *activity-selection* intervention involves therapists working with clients to identify activities that improve mood and then working with them to increase their engagement in those activities. The *skill-building* intervention involves a therapist working with a client to identify a skill she wants to develop and then helping her list and engage in the steps needed to build the skill. This module borrows from these interventions, but the focus here is distinct, emphasizing the emotion-regulation benefits of mastering a skill.

Teach

Being Good at Something Makes It Easier to Deal with Feelings

Mastery promotes emotion regulation via two processes. First, there is a *preventive* benefit: doing things you're good at can help you feel better, and feeling better helps you better handle triggers for negative feelings. Second, there is a *treatment* benefit: doing things you're good at can improve mood, even when your mood is quite low (e.g., as a result of an unwanted or unpleasant event). Therapists can emphasize both of these teaching points with clients and caregivers, soliciting examples from the family's lives or else offering examples from the therapist's own experiences.

Practice: Activities and Games

There are no games for this module. Instead, the therapist should help the client identify an activity and then create a plan to begin to build mastery with that activity. The basic sequence is: (1) select an activity, (2) schedule practice of the activity, and (3) observe the impact of the activity.

Select an Activity

The first step in guiding a client toward mastering a skill is to come up with some possible activities.

Activity Generation: Basics. Many clients will have no trouble identifying an activity at which they excel, but for those who do struggle, a good exercise can be to make a long list of a variety of activities. Such brainstorming exercises can also help a client who is stuck in the "nothing is fun anymore" mind-set. Although some therapists hesitate to make suggestions to clients, it can be quite helpful to do so, as long as the therapist listens carefully for client interest. Therapists can suggest activities that the client said he once liked, as well as ones that the therapist thinks he may like. Wise therapists avoid telling the client what to do. Instead, they offer suggestions in a curious and "scientific" manner, as if guessing or proposing a research hypothesis.

In general, it is best to hide any personal feelings about ideas offered. Furthermore, therapists are encouraged to suggest some ideas that are patently silly. By doing so, one provides a model of brainstorming that is a free-for-all activity and not one limited to "only the best ideas," thereby encouraging clients to offer their own ideas. For some clients, though, new ideas from the therapist are just what they need.

The initial goal is to create a list that includes two (or more) activities that meet *all* of the following criteria.

1. The client finds the activity enjoyable.
2. The client is permitted to engage in the activity (i.e., the caregiver approves).
3. The activity meets *at least one* of the following criteria:
   a. The client is already good at the activity and can improve.
   b. The client appears willing to develop competency in the activity.
4. The activity meets *both* of the following criteria:
   a. The activity is fun regardless of the person's skill level.
   b. The fun level of the activity is stable or increases with repetition.
5. The activity is a healthy one. For example, although video games are likely to be on many of the lists your clients generate, encouraging video game use (or watching TV and even reckless and potentially dangerous activities) is not advised.

Activity Generation: Troubleshooting. Some clients will refuse to acknowledge that any activity will be fun or will insist that they are not good at anything. Sometimes, offering a list of potential activities is all the encouragement the client needs. If not, there are a few choices.

First, a therapist may choose to move to another module. Sometimes the best ideas for interventions with clients do not work, not because they are bad interventions but because the timing is wrong or the intervention does not fit the client. If a therapist does decide to move on to "Plan B," she should select another intervention that addresses a core target already identified for the case. As would be expected, the recommendation here is to rely on the functional assessment to guide the choice (see Chapter 4).

Sometimes, though, a therapist may want to persist despite the client's resistance. Persistence can be a good choice if a therapist thinks having the client do something he is good at will make a big difference, or if the therapist thinks the client is actually interested in the activity brainstorming and is only "playing" at the resistance. The recommended cognitive stance of the therapist is *not* to assume that any particular activity will help; instead, the therapist should model curiosity about what the activity's impact will be. The case example here demonstrates a way that a therapist might work around resistance from a client, 14-year-old Steve, who has been quite depressed for nearly 7 months.

STEVE: None of that stuff on the list looks fun. And I'm not good at those things anyway.

THERAPIST: Okay. I understand. Sometimes even my favorite meal, burritos, can sound terrible. Let's do an experiment together. I have a hypothesis. You remember what a hypothesis is?

STEVE: Duh—a guess.

THERAPIST: Yep—fancy word for guess. Well, I have a guess. You see, I've worked with other kids and we have picked things from lists like this one. Then the kids have done those things a bunch of times. And you know what? Doing the activity helped for some kids. Not all kids . . . but some. My hypothesis is that it will work for you. But the only way we'll know if it works for you is to try it. And how will we know whether it works?

STEVE: Well, it won't.

THERAPIST: Let's pretend that I was working with another kid and we were trying to figure out whether it was working with that kid. How would we know whether it was working?

STEVE: You'd have to ask that kid.

THERAPIST: That's right. I might take ratings, for example. We could do an experiment to see whether the hypothesis is correct. I think we should test that hypothesis with you. I want to go through the list again, and this time let's have you mark each activity that *used to be fun* with a plus sign, like this. *(Demonstrates.)*

(Client and therapist work on sheet, marking only a few activities.)

> THERAPIST: Fantastic! Now, let's go through the list one more time, this time marking each one that you *already know how to do* with a star, like this. *(Demonstrates.)*
>
> *(Client and therapist work on sheet, marking a few activities.)*
>
> THERAPIST: Okay—here is the experiment part! We have to pick one of the activities marked with either a star or a plus sign. There are only three of them, so that should be easy.
>
> STEVE: None of those will help.
>
> THERAPIST: Sounds like you have a hypothesis too. Let's test them both. Which one of these three should we use to test our hypotheses?

Finally, it is often important to enlist a caregiver in this process. A caregiver can help generate activities for the list as well as provide support once the client is ready to begin practicing the activity.

Schedule Practice of the Activity

Once the activity has been selected, the next step is to set up a practice schedule.

Start with Success. The initial aim when scheduling is to ensure that there will be early success, such that the client feels good about her performance in the activity and also the extent of her practicing. The reasoning is simple. When many people aim for behavior change, they plan as if they were a football team losing by 20 points. They feel pressure to score a lot of points—and in a hurry. So they look for the big play to get all of those points right away, generally setting an overly ambitious goal. Such a plan can work well if the client is highly motivated and has the perseverance and support needed to meet the demands of the schedule. However, too often, a few missed practices can leave a client discouraged.

As an example, consider a client who is interested in learning how to play the drums. There may be a temptation to schedule that activity every night for 2 hours, a schedule that would certainly build competency. And for some clients, that may work just fine. But for many, the plan will be foiled because the client will not adhere to the schedule and then be tempted to say either (1) "I can't do it—I told you" or (2) "Your plan didn't work. Why should I try more of your ideas?"

Instead, the best advice is usually to start small and build from there. Sometimes success means following through on a planned activity *once*. Although doing something once may not seem like much to the client or the client's family (or perhaps to the therapist), when compared to the base rate (i.e., zero), one time is a move in the right direction. And once the "one" is established, the client can move up to "two," and so on. Helping a client and his caregivers refine their view of success to include these incremental steps is important to helping them achieve the greater success they are looking for.

Identify the What? Who? and When? Another important part of planning and scheduling is thinking through all of the obstacles to success. One helpful way to accomplish this is to walk through an examination of the What?, Who?, and When? of practicing mastery activities.

What? What exactly is meant by "practice"? Does 5 minutes count? Does it count as practicing basketball if a basketball was not involved (e.g., running sprints or distance to build stamina)? It can help to write out the "practice" as if writing out a carefully worded prescription. "Paint a picture with at least three different colors on one 8½" × 11" piece of paper." And it can also be helpful to role-play the practice to help the therapist identify any misunderstandings or misappraisals.

Who? Can the client do the activity without help? Or are others needed, like a caregiver for transportation, or a teammate or a competitor for some sports? If others are needed, the goal is to help think that through with a client, perhaps even helping make those arrangements. For example, a client can plan with the caregiver during the therapy meeting how to get to the event. Or the therapist can work with the client to line up the relevant people, even using session time to contact needed helpers by phone or e-mail.

The following therapy excerpt involves a client, Chad, introduced in Chapter 4. As a quick reminder, Chad is the 9-year-old brought in for treatment by his parents for moderate behavior problems at home and school (e.g., teasing other kids, defiance at home, tantrums).

THERAPIST: Guess what we're going to do now?

CHAD: Um, probably practice.

THERAPIST: Yep—you have a good memory for what we do in here. So, the idea is to practice swimming like we talked about before. What would that look like?

CHAD: Um, you want me to show you how to swim?

THERAPIST: *(Laughs.)* I can be a little silly, huh? Well, maybe you can show me how to swim in a minute. But right now, let's think about what the different steps are to practice swimming. So, first step?

CHAD: Well, get in the pool?

THERAPIST: For sure, you will need to get in the pool. But I'm talking about starting from your house. You don't have a pool in your house, do you?

CHAD: I wish.

THERAPIST: Okay, so what would you need to do first? Let's act this out. I will be you and you can be your mother. We are at your house. What day would be good for practice?

CHAD: Um, well. Hmm. I don't know.

THERAPIST: That can be a tough question, I know. We can ask your mom when she comes in later. But let's say just for now that a good day would be Wednesday.

CHAD: Okay. What am I supposed to do?

THERAPIST: So, I am you, you are your mother. How would I get to practice swimming? What should I do first?

CHAD: Well, you would have to ask mom to drive you to the Y.

THERAPIST: So let's try that. I am you. You be your mom.

[as Chad] Um, Mom, I think it's time to go practice swimming at the Y.

CHAD: [as mom] *(using a funny voice)* Okay, let's go.

THERAPIST: So far, so good. Now, a tricky question for you. How long is long enough for practice?

CHAD: I don't know.

THERAPIST: What makes sense to you? What do you think you can do?

CHAD: Two hours?

THERAPIST: Wow! Two hours would be great. That would be a lot of practice. Let me ask about something else real quick. Do you ever have to clean your room?

CHAD: Yeah—I hate that.

THERAPIST: Yeah—me too! One thing I have learned about cleaning my room is that I usually feel like it is going to take forever to do. So I don't do it. So what I have learned is to schedule just a little bit of cleaning, like 5 or 10 minutes. And then I stop and see how it's going. Sometimes practicing like we are talking about works that way too. So 2 hours would be awesome, but maybe less would be okay, too? And it might be easier to do. What do you think?

CHAD: Yeah—maybe. Like an hour?

THERAPIST: An hour is great! I might even suggest something less for the first time. Maybe 15 or 30 minutes. You can always do more. But once you hit 15 or 30 minutes, you can think, "I did it." And sometimes I even find that kids do great with only 10 minutes. It's like when I clean my room for 10 minutes and think, "Hmm, that wasn't so hard, and now it's half done. I bet I can get this finished quickly." When we aim small, it actually helps us do big things. Why don't we try that with this practice?

CHAD: Okay—like 15 minutes of swimming?

THERAPIST: A great place to start.

When? Identifying *when* to do the activity is as important as being clear about what the activity is. Often, a caregiver can be instrumental in identifying a good time and helping remind the client. As mentioned earlier, a therapist can pretend to use a prescription pad to specify what and when to practice, including specific days and times.

Observe the Impact of the Activity

Ratings let the client and therapist know whether the activity is helping the client improve his skills and improving the client's mood.

Kinds of Ratings. There are at least two kinds or categories of ratings that will help with this module.

- **Mood.** The goal is to determine whether the activity has influenced mood, so some rating is helpful. There is no magic to the actual scale one chooses. Many therapists opt for a traditional 0–10 scale, where 10 means "very happy" and 0 means "very depressed." A smaller range of scores may be useful for younger clients. And there is no need to use numbers at all, at least not with the client herself. Some therapists use a range of faces to reflect a scale; others use a range of colors. These non-numeric scales can be converted into numbers, of course, and doing so is often useful, as the scores can be graphed to show the client progress (or lack thereof).
- **Mastery.** A second important rating is mastery. Here the goal is to gauge how "well" the client is performing the activity. Again, the scaling can run the gamut from traditional 0–10 to picture or color ratings. The therapeutic hope, of course, is that the scale will show gradual increases over time.
- **Other scales.** Of course, there are other possible ratings to take during the activities associated with this module. Some therapists have used "fun," "people are noticing me in a good way," and "want to do it again" ratings, as a few examples. Therapists are encouraged to tailor the rating process to the client's strengths and needs.

Timing of Ratings. Taking "before" and "after" (and sometimes "during") ratings is a way to know whether an intervention is producing the desired effect. It is recommended to use at least pre/post ratings on a regular basis. Some clients may refuse to give ratings or may give ratings that therapists do not think are optimally valid. In such cases, caregivers can be involved in the monitoring process.

What If Ratings Do Not Improve? If the ratings do not increase, then the therapist should assess why. Perhaps the activity does not actually make the client feel better. Or perhaps it does, but inconsistently, or only after a few repetitions. Also, the client may not want the therapist (or caregiver) to know that the activity has an impact. A collaborative empiricist approach can be quite helpful in exploring why an intervention may not be yielding the expected results: "Let's do some experiments to see what works. We may have to try this a few times to understand it better. And some of the ideas we try will not work. Every person is a little different. But we will keep trying until we find something."

Therapists are encouraged to use these ratings as one basis for changing the course of the treatment. It may be that the activity chosen was not the best one for the purposes here. Alternatively, it may be that helping the client experience mastery has a negligible benefit for him. Without ratings, the therapist could only guess about the effects of the intervention. With ratings, the therapist can use the data to adjust or change course.

MODULE 6

Emotion Regulation Skills III
Expression Skills

This is the first of the three emotion regulation modules designed to bolster emotion regulation "in the moment." It focuses on ways to teach clients to express their feelings in difficult situations to maximize their adaptation to those situations. (For antecedent management strategies, see Modules 4 and 5.)

WHEN TO USE THIS MODULE

This module is designed for use when a major contributor to a client's difficulties is a lack of skills in regulating emotions *specifically related to emotional expression*. The client might not express her feelings, at least not out loud to anyone. Or perhaps the client does express her feelings, but in a way that interferes with functioning (e.g., by sharing so often that others tire of the constant expression). Cases at both extremes are well served by this module.

OBJECTIVES

Objectives for this module are to teach and practice ways to express emotional experience, with the "proposed" outcome being (1) that things will be "better" (i.e., easier, more manageable) and (2) that the feelings, once expressed, will be less intense and/or less troubling. The strategies described in this module are not focused on any specific feeling. Instead, they are designed to apply to most if not all emotions.

The module focuses on two different sets of strategies for teaching emotional expression skills. The first focus is on starting and/or increasing the quantity (and to some extent, the quality) of emotional expression. The second focus is on helping clients optimize their emotional expression (i.e., quality improvement.) That is, the first focus is for clients who have limited emotional expression skills, and the second is for clients who express their emotions, but often in problematic ways. Therapists may target one or the other foci (or both), as warranted by the case conceptualization.

PROCEDURES

Step 1. Regulating Emotion: An Introduction

If Step 1 from Module 4 has not already been covered with the client, the therapist can use material from it as an introduction to the utility of emotion regulation. If therapists have already covered the material, though, there is no need to repeat it unless client could benefit from the review.

Step 2. Expressing Yourself

Overview

Expressing emotions is an important emotion regulation strategy that is *underappreciated* and subject to being called *trite*. "Tell me how you feel about that . . ." is perhaps *the* stereotypical therapist line. Learning how to express (and control expression) of emotions is an important developmental achievement, but there is a lot of misunderstanding about why and how therapists encourage clients of all ages to express their feelings.

Teach

Expressing Feelings Makes It Easier to Deal with Those Feelings

Feelings Tell You What Matters. As discussed in Chapter 2, emotions are (ideally) functional insofar as they "notify" a person that an event "matters" in a personal way. For example, imagine that Sam and Eli are good friends. If they are playing together at Sam's house and then Eli leaves, Sam might feel sad. That feeling tells Sam how important Eli is to him. If Sam instead felt relieved in the same situation, the feeling would tell a different story about his relationship with Eli.

For many clients, hearing that their feelings do not reflect deep-seated problems but, rather, are their bodies' way of reminding them what is important can be a relief. Having troublesome feelings can be viewed as inconvenient, annoying, or even some indicator of being "crazy." To replace these messages, the therapist can assure the client that feelings are legitimate. In fact, feelings are allies. They teach people what is important to them, what they value. So listening to feelings is important.

Reflect on What It Is That Matters, Because, Well, It Matters. Not all feelings are created equal. Rampant, indiscriminate sharing of feelings can be problematic. Many therapists have observed clients whose oversharing hurts others (e.g., providing less than constructive feedback in the name of expressing oneself) or whose tendency to emote constantly pushes others away or makes it difficult for others to share their own feelings and experiences. Before expressing feelings, it helps to reflect on what exactly matters. There are a few dimensions to consider and discuss with the client.

Who (or What) Is the Presumed "Target" of the Feelings? Here, a therapist helps a client identify the person toward whom the feeling is being felt. In other words, you are feeling sad "about" (or "toward") which person(s)? It is important to remember that the target can be the client herself. It is also important to keep in mind that the true target can sometimes be denied or hidden. Here is a personal example: Driving in moderate traffic, I start feeling frustrated. I may reason that the car in front of me is the true target of the frustration because it is going so slowly and I am running late. However, upon reflection, I may see that I am frustrated with myself too because I was late leaving the house. As the example makes clear, a feeling can (and often does) have more than one target.

What Is the Presumed "Reason" for the Feeling? Here, the therapist and client grapple with the big "why?" question, as in "Why am I so angry?" Again, there are often multiple reasons—and not all are easy to admit. Many times, the easiest reasons to identify are those that are someone else's "fault." As noted in Module 2, understanding the "external" causes of emotions comes before understanding the internal reasons. Furthermore, it is easier to give reasons that are *acceptable*—to our perspective on the situation, to our family's culture, or to the culture in which one is being raised. Giving those *other* reasons, those that may be obscured by pride, culture, or both, requires courage and thought.

To use another personal example, I sometimes become frustrated when my children have not finished their homework on time. I can tell myself and them I am frustrated because I have mentioned the homework several times and they know they are supposed to do it. Thus their failure to complete the homework is one reason I am frustrated—and an obvious and easy one to admit. However, I may also be angry for a variety of other reasons, including (1) if the homework is not done, we will be delayed in the next activity (one that perhaps I am interested in); (2) I could or should have used a different strategy in helping or guiding the homework; or (3) the failure to complete the homework may mean something "bad" about my kids.

In short, there are many reasons for feelings to arise. The more one understands them, the better one will be able to deal with one's feelings. And knowing about the more embarrassing reasons for certain feelings may be particularly important.

There are a few other points that therapists may want to consider making in relation to the broader point of becoming more aware of one's feelings and the reasons one is experiencing them.

- **Each reason can lead to its own feelings trajectory.** Each reason for the feeling has implications for how long one may experience that feeling as well as what other feelings may occur as a result of the initial feeling.
- **People can have feelings about things that are only imagined or forecasted.** A feeling can arise due to events that have not (and may not ever) come to pass. So the search for reasons for feelings must delve into clients' thoughts and predictions and not just in the events of the day.
- **People can have feelings that are completely tied to past events over which they have no control.** Thus the past is also a place to search for the reasons for feelings.
- **Some reasons for feelings may seem petty or unimportant.** People may feel hurt or upset in situations that, when carefully and honestly considered, seem silly. The therapist's job in such cases is not to agree with the client about the ridiculousness of the feeling. Instead, the therapist should note the humanity and normalcy of such a feeling and gently move to discussing the fact that one need not act on all feelings.
- **The reasons clients hide the most strongly may be the most salient.** Sometimes, gains in treatment are observed only when the hidden reasons see the light of day, to be expressed and evaluated. For example, take the client whose frequent anger, generally blamed on other people, is suddenly traced to anxiety, a fear that the client's mother is going to leave him. The hidden reason for anger, a fear of abandonment, warrants discussion.

Sometimes, thinking through the reasons for feelings will lead a client to consider changes in interpersonal relationships (as reflected in the next step). In other instances, the reason review may lead to changes in how the client thinks about things, a point returned to in Modules 7 and 8.

Feelings Are Meant to Be Shared

Emotions are interpersonal events as much as they are intrapersonal ones. Sharing feelings, even unpleasant ones, is often good for relationships. However, as noted, sharing *all feelings, all the time* is not beneficial. Instead, one has to know which to share, when to share, and how to share.

Which Feelings to Share? The initial aim with many clients is to get the spigot turned on—that is, to get the client to share any feelings at all. Once the spigot is on, the therapist can model and practice how he might think through which feelings to share, using real and hypothetical situations. The following case example provides some idea of how this can work in a session. Here, the client is Meredith, a 12-year-old with social anxiety and moderate depression.

THERAPIST: Let's try this out. Say you are at your best friend's birthday party and you taste the food and it's awful. Good time to express your feelings?

MEREDITH: Um, well, no. I mean, I wouldn't eat much, but I don't think I should say anything. That might be rude.

THERAPIST: Makes sense. What if you really liked the food?

MEREDITH: Oh, definitely say something.

THERAPIST: Good. Now let's make it a bit more challenging. Let's say you tried out for a play at your school, and so did your good friend. Let's say you got the part and she did not. How would you feel?

MEREDITH: Um, happy. Maybe proud, too. But I would feel bad for her, I think.

THERAPIST: Yeah—good. So what would you express?

MEREDITH: Oh, well. Hmm. I'm not sure. I guess I might not say anything to her. Like, she might not want to talk about it.

THERAPIST: Yeah—that is one way to do it. What if she said to you, "Congratulations"?

MEREDITH: Oh, well, I might say, "Thanks." And then maybe say something like, "I got lucky."

THERAPIST: Oh, I see. Like, downplay your feelings?

MEREDITH: Yeah, I guess. I mean, it might hurt her feelings to act happy.

THERAPIST: Great work. Now let's try one more. In this one, let's say your friend Sandy got in trouble for breaking the rules at home. And so she is grounded.

MEREDITH: Bad one.

THERAPIST: Yep. And Sandy's mom took her cell phone away and won't let her get on the computer at all. So Sandy already told her mom that she thinks it's unfair and that she's angry about these punishments. Now let's say that later in the day, Sandy is still feeling mad about it. Do you think she should share her feelings with her mom again?

MEREDITH: Hmm. Well, probably not.

THERAPIST: Why not?

MEREDITH: I don't know, seems like a bad idea.

THERAPIST: Why? What makes it a bad idea? She is feeling mad, right? And telling our feelings to people is a sometimes a good idea, right?

MEREDITH: Yeah, I guess, but . . . I don't think it would help anything.

THERAPIST: What might happen?

MEREDITH: Her mom might get mad at her.

THERAPIST: Oh, right. That is a good point. Hmm, what might happen to Sandy's feelings?

MEREDITH: If she shared again? I don't know.

THERAPIST: Let's think it through. Let's say she tells her mom she is still mad and her mom gets a little annoyed with her. Then how will Sandy feel?

MEREDITH: I think that might make her feel worse. They will probably yell at each other.

When To Share? Many young children say what they want, when they want, sometimes to the inconvenience of others. With age comes a new perspective: that other people have feelings of their own and will respond differently depending on their own moods and situations. A child may learn that her mother is pretty good at hearing what she has to say when she is driving but that talking while driving makes her father irritable. To learn to what extent a client is already privy to this sort of knowledge, the following questions can help:

---

1. When would be the BEST/WORST time to ask your mom/dad/care-giver for money?

2. When would be the BEST/WORST time to tell your mom/dad/care-giver you got into trouble?

3. When would be the BEST/WORST time to tell your mom/dad/care-giver about some good news like a good grade on a test?

4. When would be the BEST/WORST time to tell your mom/dad/care-giver that you have a new friend at school?

How to Share? This refers not only to body language and voice tone, but also to the medium. Some clients will express feelings most readily by talking. Others will feel more comfortable with writing. Still others prefer to draw or use art. Even within one of these categories, there are many possible variations. For instance, some clients will talk about their feelings when directly asked, one on one. Other clients will be more willing to share their feelings when engaged in some other activity like playing a game or tossing a ball. Therapists can use session time to describe and rehearse these different ways of sharing feelings to see which fits each client best. In the end, though, the goal is for the client to find some way to share his feelings with significant others in his life. To do so, most often the client will need to learn how to talk about feelings. Although practicing emotional expression in session using multiple modalities is encouraged, therapists will need to guide the client to practice talking with others about his feelings.

Practice: Activities and Games

The obvious and stereotypical therapy line—that talking about your feelings is a good thing—can ring hollow to many clients. So helping clients understand the value of this point can be challenging. Another challenge is that therapists are trained to receive almost anything a client can say with equal amounts of understanding, empathy, support, and affirmation—in addition to rarely if ever seeming surprised or offended (most therapists have heard everything!). In a sense, therapists are as "perfect" at listening as humans can be, and so do have that working in their favor with clients who are reluctant to share. Obviously, though, the plan is not for the therapist to move in with the client and become his confidant. Accordingly, the goal here is to help the client identify other trusted people with whom to share his feelings. For both challenges there is a need to practice.

The good news is that there are myriad ways to help clients express their feelings. Here are three specific activities that have an evidence base to support their use and are flexible in their use across a number of age ranges and problem areas.

Walking the Talk

The following activity often occurs across several meetings. The four steps answer the questions "who," "what," "why," and "how."

To Whom Can You Talk? This step can be as simple as creating a list of people with whom the client is comfortable or willing to share his feelings. The list can be constructed as a hierarchy, including some people with whom discussing feelings would be relatively easy as well as other people with whom the task would be a challenge but with whom the benefits of the discussion are potentially strong (at least by the therapist's judgment). For example, a client may not initially put her parents on the list. The therapist is encouraged to add the parents' names, assuming the therapist views the parents as viable listeners (i.e., not unchangeably abusive). The therapist can offer the caveat that although the client is not presently open to the idea, the therapist has known many clients for whom that changes over time. Thus the therapist makes discussions with the parent into a possibility, one open to empirical testing.

So how to create this list? The therapist's job, as always, is to provide not answers but ideas. A list of possible folks with whom to share feelings does not contain any "must haves." Each option is a question, not a mandate. The therapist can ask, "I wonder how it would go to talk with person X?" Therapists can be handy in offering those less likely candidates, like extended family members, teachers, coaches, and religious leaders. Ideally, the goal is to create a list of people who together (i.e., not individually, necessarily, but as a group) meet *all* of the following criteria.

1. Easily accessible
2. High likelihood of support
3. A person with whom the therapist can occasionally speak
4. High likelihood of positive modeling (i.e., will give good advice and support the client's growth and adaptive choices)

What Are You Going to Talk about? The next step is to generate a list of feelings topics to discuss with the people on the list. This process can be akin to creating a fear hierarchy when conducting exposure therapy for anxiety. The therapist and client collaborate on building a list of topics that generate emotions. With the list in hand, the therapist then creates a hierarchy of sorts, taking ratings of the difficulty in discussing those feelings with people on the list, keeping in mind that the ratings may differ by topic and person. Examples of topics would range from feelings the client has about schoolwork to feelings about different classmates or family members, with the specific feelings themselves ranging across the whole gamut.

Why Is It Important to Talk? The third step is to remind the client why talking about her feelings is useful. Specifically, therapists will want to discuss talking about feelings for emotional support and/or instrumental support. Here, each is discussed each briefly, as the two are distinct.

Emotional Support. Sometimes all someone needs is a witness for his feelings: "I hear ya!" or "That stinks!" or "Great news!" It can be helpful for therapists to make clear to clients (and the list of potential listeners) that sometimes emotional expression is just that—expression of a momentary feeling and not a cause for some major action. Clients should know that it is normal to want their feelings heard and empathized with, without anything else happening. Some clients may be concerned that by sharing their feelings they will be forced to have long discussions and then have to "solve" the problem(s) associated with the feeling. Therapists can assure clients (and their family members) that in some situations, simply being heard is all that "talking about feelings" has to involve. It can be as simple as the client saying, "I felt really lonely today because I did not see my friend Jessica," followed by the listener saying something as simple as, "Being lonely is not very fun. I hope you see Jessica again soon" or even, "Bummer."

Instrumental Support. Sometimes feelings identify important problems that do warrant action, of course, as if the feelings are saying, "This problem needs some solution!" This is common across all developmental stages (even throughout adulthood, obviously), but it is especially noticeable with younger children because they often need someone to help them navigate the complicated world of emotions, particularly when the causes are interpersonal situations. The kind of support needed can range from problem-solving advice to actual actions taken on behalf of the client.

How Do You Talk about Feelings?

Time and Place. Earlier in the module, the issue of timing was discussed in the context of gauging a client's sense of the best and worst times to mention specific topics with adults. The basic notion to discuss with the client here is to "pick your spots" when talking about feelings. Therapists who excel at this step often have a good set of examples at their fingertips to use in a quick game in which a situation is described and then the following question is asked: "Is this a good time to let the person know that you feel *X*?" where *X* is a feeling.

Feeling + Reason = Expressing Yourself. This is a familiar construction for most therapists. Expressing a feeling involves naming the feeling and explaining why the feeling is there. The "reasons" are often complicated and therapists are sometimes tempted to engage in overprocessing of the feeling. In the beginning, though, it may be best to generate just one reason for the feeling. Over time and with practice, therapists can shape the client's understanding of and appreciation for "other" reasons. As a simple example, a client might say: "I feel angry because the teacher yelled at me." A more nuanced statement would be: "I feel angry because I was embarrassed in front of others when the teacher yelled at me." An advanced statement might be: "I feel angry because I care what others think, and I worry now that others think less of me because the teacher yelled at me for something I did wrong." In the beginning, the first statement is the goal. Over time, therapists can work toward eliciting the more advanced examples.

Optional: Feeling + Reason + Request = Expressing Yourself. The optional step here is adding a request, which is essentially asking for what one thinks one needs because of a certain feeling. For some clients, being able to understand and then communicate whether they are seeking instrumental or emotional support helps them get the help they need.

The following case example shows a therapist walking a client through the "how" steps of talking about feelings. The client is Brittney, the 14-year-old described in some detail in Chapter 4, who tends to ruminate on upsetting situations.

THERAPIST: Now we're going to practice, just like usual. You already said that this is a little different than how you usually do it, so why don't I do the hard part first? You can be the person listening and I will tell you about an upsetting feeling that I'm having.

BRITTNEY: What do I do?

THERAPIST: Great question—we haven't really said what the listener does! Listening is a hard job, really. Why don't we make this easy? You just listen and then when I am done, tell me back what you heard, as best as you can.

BRITTNEY: Okay. I listen to my friend Greg all the time.

THERAPIST: Right, so here I go. I will be a 15-year-old girl, a sophomore in high school. And let's say I had a bad day at school and I come home in a funk. You can be my mom, so that would be the "who?" step. *(Gestures at the list of possible listeners constructed earlier in the session.)* And my crummy day, that will be the "what?" The next step . . . ?

BRITTNEY: Um, . . . the "why?" So, why are you going to tell me, right?

THERAPIST: Right, great! Okay, and last . . . ?

BRITTNEY: The "how?" These are really kinda obvious.

THERAPIST: And how should I do this?

BRITTNEY: You just tell me, like, your feeling and then . . . the reason you feel that way.

THERAPIST: Perfect! That's right. And one more thing—before we do this, we always . . . ?

BRITTNEY: The ratings, right. Who gives a rating? You?

THERAPIST: Yeah. We'll see what happens to my rating when I tell you how I'm feeling. So, let's say I'm coming home and my mood rating is a 3 out of 10.

BRITTNEY: Low. Bummer.

THERAPIST: Okay, here we go.

THERAPIST: (as teen) Hey, Mom. Um *(long pause)*.

BRITTNEY: You have a lot of homework tonight?

THERAPIST: (as teen) Yeah, but, um, I am in a bad mood right now because of something that happened at school.

BRITTNEY: You have a lot of homework tonight?

THERAPIST: (as teen) Well, yeah, but . . .

BRITTNEY: Spill it.

THERAPIST: (*Laughs.*) Very funny, Brittney! I guess I am having trouble telling how I feel. Let me give it a try.
   [as teen] Um, at school I felt sad because Emma was making fun of me, calling me a prude, for my outfit. *(breaking character)* Wow! That was kinda hard. How did I do?

BRITTNEY: Good.

THERAPIST: Let's go through the steps. *What* and *who*. How did I do there?

BRITTNEY: Good—you told me, I mean your mom, and you told me about Emma making fun of your outfit.

THERAPIST: Right. What's next?

BRITTNEY: Um, oh right—why? You didn't really do that one.

> THERAPIST: You're right. I wonder why I would tell you about the thing with Emma?
>
> BRITTNEY: Girls making fun of you? Well, definitely not to get your mom to do something. That would be a bad idea.
>
> THERAPIST: Good—so one reason would be to get help. What is other reason? Rhymes with *fort.*
>
> BRITTNEY: Um, oh, right, support. To get support. Yeah, that might be what you wanted.
>
> THERAPIST: Last step?
>
> BRITTNEY: How.
>
> THERAPIST: And how did I do there?
>
> BRITTNEY: You got that one pretty good. You told me you felt sad and you told me why.
>
> THERAPIST: Great! Now, your turn . . .

Write It Down

For clients who shy from verbal communication, putting thoughts on paper is a strategy worth trying. Writing interventions have been tested in a variety of populations, ranging from those with physical health problems (e.g., HIV, cancer, arthritis) to mental health problems (e.g., depression, trauma), with positive benefits demonstrated across a number of studies. The following recommendations provide some guidance for structuring written expression of emotion. There are some clients for whom neither verbal nor written communication will come easily. The end of this activity lists some alternative strategies.

Identify Where to Store the Writings. Spiral notebooks or composition books are good options for clients who prefer to write on paper. Clients may also choose to write on a computer or other electronic device, in which case digital documents will serve just as well. If these digital documents will be e-mailed, password protection of the documents is strongly encouraged, as is the omission of identifying information in the documents. Another alternative is to make audio or video recordings, similar to podcasting or videocasting. Research on writing interventions has not found that the modality of expression makes a difference, so go with whatever medium makes the client most comfortable.

Provide Instructions for the Task. Therapists may (and should) change the following basic instructions to adapt to the client's progress and/or needs.

What to Write. Developers of writing interventions have used a variety of options in their work. The following are the standard instructions:

> "Please write about your feelings and thoughts about a **significant and upsetting event.** It is important that when you are writing you really let go and explore your feelings and thoughts about the event as honestly as you can."

Here are some (and not exhaustive) variations that can be used for the **bolded** phrase. Readers will identify and find value in many other options.

" . . . **the most upsetting experience of your life.**"
" . . . **the most traumatic experience of your life.**"
" . . . **an upsetting recent experience.**"
" . . . **a significant and positive, happy experience.**"

Readers will note the difference in the last variation. Although most of the writing interventions focus on clients writing about upsetting events, some studies have used positive events. Data suggest that the valence of the event may not matter. In general, though, many will find it more useful to have clients writing about negative events, as these are the ones they are more likely to misappraise and ruminate about. However, for clients whose focus makes Eeyore or Lemony Snicket seem like bastions of optimism, the positive prompt can be helpful and instructive (e.g., is the client able/willing to reflect on positive events?).

The following "plug-ins" may be helpful add-ons to vary the experience as the writing work proceeds.

- **Plug-in 1: Feelings change.** This plug-in is particularly useful for clients who tend to become mired in the belief that their bad feelings will last forever. The standard instructions are used, followed by this prompt:

"After you have written an entry, put it away for at least 15 minutes. After that time, go back and read the entry again. Circle sections of the writing that seem to express the feelings more strongly than you feel them now, 15 minutes later."

For this plug-in, the therapist can also add the following instruction:

"For each circled or underlined part, write down why you think the feeling has become less intense."

This secondary instruction makes even clearer to clients that feelings can become less intense over time. Although the therapist can directly explain that fact to clients, having the client experience firsthand that "lessening" of emotion can be helpful, particularly for those who tend to be emotionally reactive.

- **Plug-in 2: Thought crimes.** This plug-in is useful for clients whose thoughts are strongly influenced by their feelings. The standard instruction is followed by the following prompt:

"After you have written an entry, put it away for at least 15 minutes. After that time, go back and read the entry again. Circle or underline any thoughts you wrote down that seem like exaggerations or seem like a time when you were focusing only on one negative aspect of the situation."

In addition, the therapist can add the following instruction:

"For each circled or underlined part, write down two different thoughts: one that would make you feel even worse and one that might make you feel better."

This prompt is helpful for clients who have trouble identifying more positive thoughts. One can take this prompt even further by adding the following:

"Rewrite the entry as if your thoughts about the situation helped you remain calm and helped you cope well."

To take this plug-in even further, one can request two versions: one that is pure fantasy, with anything allowed (e.g., magic, mythical animals), and a more realistic re-rendering of the situation. The two versions could be written sequentially, with a brief break or even no break in between. The notion with the "anything goes" version is to tap into the client's creativity. Also, the fantastic version can sometimes provide a glimpse into the client's wishes and/or hopes about the topic.

• **Plug-in 3: Alternate realities.** This plug-in is useful for clients who have trouble seeing alternative ways to deal with the challenges they experience or who have a tendency to remain stuck on the same solution to problems. The prompt is a bit different than in the first two plug-ins. Here, the client returns to a previous entry to conduct the work, rather than working from a new entry.

"Go back to a past entry. List three different ways you could have coped with your strong feelings in the situation described, if it had happened again. Next, write an entry as if one of your alternatives had indeed happened."

The idea with this plug-in is not just to list the possible ways of coping (many clients can do that). A benefit of writing is that one can ask the client to think through the pros and cons of different coping approaches, perhaps increasing the odds that the client will try one of these approaches in real life. Through the process of imagining having coped differently with a feeling, the client may begin to see the value in foregoing old coping habits. For this plug-in, modeling the process is often useful, as many clients will struggle if asked to go solo.

• **Plug-in 4: Where is the silver lining?** This plug-in is useful for clients who may benefit from seeing how even bad or challenging experiences can help them grow stronger:

> "At the end of your entry, write down one positive thing that could happen as a result of the event you are writing about."

It is worth noting that using this prompt should be done with some caution, as not all events have easily identified silver linings and there are some events, such as abuse, that are best considered wholly negative.

How Long to Write. There have been no systematic studies examining how long the writing period should be. However, most studies have used a 15- or 20-minute time period. Therapists are encouraged to start small, especially if the client has hesitations about how difficult the task will be. A sample instruction relevant to *how long* is:

> "Please write for 15 minutes. During that entire time, do your best to keep writing. Remember that there is no 'right' way to do this and that you don't need to be concerned with grammar or spelling."

How Often to Write. There have been studies designed to determine how often a person should write: several times a week or once a week or once a month? However, the results of a meta-analysis of 146 studies (Frattaroli, 2006) suggest that frequency does not matter. Thus the best current guidance is to fit the schedule to the client's needs and habits.

A relevant consideration is how many times the client should write before the therapist reads and provides feedback on the work. A good rule of thumb may be to allow one or two initial writing periods and then have a session during which those samples are discussed. That way, the therapist can adjust the client's efforts so that the benefits of the intervention are maximized. Also, having fewer writing periods between therapy sessions allows the therapist to more closely tailor the writing experience by providing frequent feedback and adding plug-ins to the prompt. For some clients, that level of therapist involvement will be useful. Other clients, especially those who appear to be benefiting from the experience, may be able to increase the frequency of their writing periods once the therapist has pointed them in the right direction.

When to Write. Therapists are encouraged to brainstorm with clients about when they will have the time, privacy, and equipment needed to complete a writing session. Therapists can encourage clients to experiment with time of day or day of the week to see how those factors influence their writing.

Remember the Purpose of Writing as an Intervention. In the beginning, encouraging any writing is the idea—the goal is to get the pump primed. Once the client has started writing, additional structure can help give the exercise direction.

Although writing *almost* anything is better than writing nothing, using the exercise only to "vent" feelings or catalogue events unemotionally is not particularly useful. Instead, the goal is to help clients connect feelings with thoughts and events and then to consider the many "angles" of a particular situation. Writing work can be a place to relive events emotionally and then construct solutions—even fantasy ones.

The therapist's role in reading the work is to help the client practice the teaching points from Step 2: (1) learning what the feeling(s) tell the client about what is important to her, (2) learning which feelings require further attention and which can be disregarded as fleeting, and (3) understanding that sharing feelings with others can be helpful. Regarding this last point, therapists are encouraged to work with clients to identify significant others in the clients' lives who might also read the writing.

Caveats and Cautionary Statements. When using writing interventions, it is important to recall that clients with emotion expression problems can have *too much* expression and/or rumination over emotions. Although the "output" of writing interventions will often focus on difficult events, there is a fine line between an appropriate focus and an overfocus. It would not be productive for the writing time to become yet another way for the client to engage in a ruminative process. There are a few ways to prevent this.

First, as noted, the therapist will be reading the entries. Once the client is engaged in the writing process, gentle feedback and Socratic consideration of the costs and benefits of the negative focus should be used. Furthermore, if problems persist, the therapist can provide additional structure to the writing. For example, co-opting the so-called "four-column" approach from cognitive therapy, a therapist can create a plug-in that involves the client writing in the following format:

---

1. Describe the situation.

2. Describe the feelings you were experiencing.

3. List the thoughts you were having.

4. List some thoughts you could have (or did have) that would have helped you feel differently (better).

The case of J.T., a 16-year-old depressed boy, demonstrates how one therapist was able to help adapt the writing intervention.

THERAPIST: Terrific work on your journal entries this week. I really like how you are putting your feelings into words. Some of these descriptions are very vivid. You know, I can see them like a movie. Great job! I also noticed that both entries were focused on Emma and Camille giving you a hard time about your having a crush on Camille.

J.T.: Yeah—that really sucked!

THERAPIST: Yeah, it sounds like it. I had an idea to try that might be a different way to do the journal. Let's use your entry from yesterday as an example. I'm going to write this out in a different way, keeping most of what you wrote and just changing a few things. Let's see if you can tell what is different *(writing while talking)*. Okay, first we'll write that Emma texted you that Camille liked you. And then we'll write that you texted back that Camille was cute, even though you didn't know her well. Any changes so far?

J.T.: Nope.

THERAPIST: Okay, good. Next I'll write that you saw Emma showing what you think was your text to other people, and they started to laugh and look at you in the lunchroom. Next, I'll write about your feelings and thoughts about that event—how angry you were, how embarrassed you felt. So far, any differences in what I am doing and what you did?

J.T.: Nope.

THERAPIST: So, after you wrote about how angry you were and how you hated those girls, you started guessing how things would go. You remember?

J.T.: Yeah, I think so. You mean when I wrote that I would never have a girlfriend at school?

THERAPIST: That's it. I will write that down too. No change there. But I am going to add one thing. And I will need your help to do it. Let's take this guess you had here, where you wrote *(reading from J.T.'s notebook)*, "Those girls were talking about what a loser I am." We're going to do two things with that statement. First, we'll write about how true we each think it is. This will be like math class because we'll have to show our work. I mean, we will have to have proof and show *why* we think it's true or not true. Second, we'll make at least one other guess about what they might have been saying, a guess that is different from the one you made but that fits with the facts we have. *(pause)* I know that is a lot, so let's go one at a time. Here is a sheet of paper for you. I will work on this one. So first, let's write down whether we think the guess you made is true—and then list out the evidence we have for our answer. Remember that the sentence is, "Those girls were talking about what a loser I am." Shall we do that aloud together or you want to do it silently?

J.T.: Silently is better.

THERAPIST: Sounds good. We can compare notes after we work at it for a few minutes. Okay, let's start.

Notice here that the therapist does not suggest that the "negative" content of the client's journal should be replaced with highly positive statements. Indeed, the journal should be a place for the client to share upsetting experiences. Instead, the therapist has begun to shape how the client can use the journal as a place to do some constructive work with those experiences.

Alternatives to the Written Word. As noted at the outset, some clients will not be keen on writing or talking. Here are a few alternative ways to teach and practice emotional expression.

Art Journal. Using art as part of therapy has a long history in mental health. Indeed, many of the instructions listed under the "writing interventions" structure could apply to an art journal that uses drawings, paintings, etc. to express feelings and thoughts about particular events.

As with a written journal, the focus should not be creativity for its own sake. Instead, the goal is to guide clients toward a means of expressing their feelings (and related thoughts) in a way that promotes a broader understanding of the situation and their feelings. In addition, the goal is to increase the client's competency in expressing those feelings. Instructions might include: "Next time, draw the situation as if a different outcome had occurred, a more positive outcome." Or, "You really included a lot of important detail here. I love how you used colors to express your feelings. Next, I would like you to paint the same scene, except this time imagine you could change how you behaved. Paint it so we can see the differences that would make."

Although drawing and painting lend themselves to this work most easily, some therapists will find ways to make other media work well.

Photo Slideshow, Audio Podcast, or Video Journal. Some clients respond well to making what amounts to a photo or video blog that serves the same purposes as the writing interventions described earlier, and the same standard instructions can be given as with the writing intervention. Examples include:

- A photo slideshow that describes or expresses the client's feelings and thoughts about a troubling situation.
- A video or audio recording of the client talking about a difficult situation.

Performance Journal. Some clients are born performers and may find expressing themselves easier in a performance, like a song or even a brief play. A performance approach lends itself well to having alternative takes or versions, making the revision and shaping work somewhat easier. The therapist can use a film metaphor with clients even when not using this specific intervention because it allows the therapist to provide feedback on the production with impunity (e.g., "Let's take that one from the top. But this time let's see if you can change how that last part goes, when you wound up arguing with your stepmom. Try it differently so the character doesn't end up arguing.")

Suggesting a new ending does not, of course, mean suggesting that the client adopt the attitude of Pollyanna, that optimistic character from Eleanor Porter's early 20th-century novel. Instead, the goal is to work with the client to cocreate reasonable and realistic alternatives, in part to demonstrate that such outcomes can be possible.

To Share or Not to Share

The final game described here is designed primarily for those clients whose quantity of emotional expression is probably too high. For such clients, the therapist will want to emphasize that sharing feelings all the time can lead to a number of negative outcomes, such as an overfocus on one's emotional state as well as possible alienation of friends. The following game can help clients who tend to provide too much information (TMI) by promoting two separate but related skills: editing emotion talk and changing the channel.

Preparation. The therapist should have a copy of the **To Share or Not to Share (Handout 1)** (or something similar) available for the client. In addition, the therapist will need to create a set of scenarios, written on index cards. Each scenario should involve a person who has a choice about whether to tell others about the emotion he or she is experiencing. The most useful set of cards will include various emotions and emotion intensities. Some examples are included here, although most therapists will want to create their own set of cards.

Scenario 1: Traci is angry at her mother, who has taken away a privilege (e.g., cell phone, media time) because Traci broke a house rule (was late, did not complete chore). It is Saturday. Traci told her mother she was upset in the morning, but now it's dinner time and she still feels really angry.

Scenario 2: Tyler's girlfriend, Trixie, broke up with him 2 months ago. Tyler has been very sad since then and shares his sadness verbally with whomever will listen. His best friend, Troy, and a few other pals are going to a concert together. On the car ride there, Tyler is feeling very sad about Trixie.

Scenario 3: Teri is at an amusement park with her class. Teri is very fearful of heights. She notices that her group is approaching a tall rollercoaster, with many of her classmates talking excitedly about how cool the ride is supposed to be. Teri is very afraid about going on the rollercoaster. She remembers a story about someone who was badly hurt on a rollercoaster, although it may not have been this particular one.

Gameplay. With the **To Share or Not to Share** handout and situation cards in hand, gameplay is quite simple. The first player draws a situation card and reads it.

Then the player reviews the "Editing Emotion Talk" guidelines from the handout, discussing each in relation to the situation. Then the player makes a choice: share or don't share. If the player chooses "share," the scene is role-played, with the first player acting as the situation's primary character and the second player taking on any other roles in the situation. If the player chooses "don't share," the player consults "Changing the Emotional Channel" guidelines from the handout, identifies the strategy he will use in this situation, and then role-plays that outcome.

After the role play, the second player provides feedback to the first player (primary character) on how he handled the situation.

The therapist may choose to modify the game such that after the situation is role-played in the mode chosen (i.e., share or don't share), the players repeat the role play using the opposite mode.

To Share or Not to Share

Editing Emotion Talk

✓ **Has the feeling already been shared?** Sharing feelings does not mean repeating them multiple times. Sometimes, saying how you feel once can be enough.

✓ **Can the feeling wait to be shared?** The real question is not, "Can *I* wait to share?" but rather, "Does the feeling need to be shared *right now* or else something truly bad will happen?"

✓ **Does the feeling need to be shared?** Not all feelings need to be shared. Be selective. Let fleeting feelings pass. It can be useful to ask, "What do I hope will happen when I share the feeling?"

✓ **Will sharing the feeling help the situation?** Do you think that sharing will improve the situation for you and others?

Changing the Emotional Channel

✓ **Do something active.** Distraction can be a helpful way to deal with a feeling you want to share but have decided you shouldn't, at least not at the moment. Doing something active (e.g., going for a run or walk, playing ball, or riding a bike) can get your body moving and pull attention away from the feeling.

✓ **Do something helpful or constructive.** Do a chore, clean out a drawer, rake the leaves—any activity that will be helpful or constructive.

✓ **Do something creative.** Make some art, sing, dance.

Emotion Regulation Skills IV
Basic Cognitive Skills

The final two modules focus on using cognitive strategies as a means for emotion regulation. Cognitive strategies are one example of what emotion scientists call *effortful regulation* strategies. As such, they represent developmentally advanced ways to deal with feelings that children encounter in their daily lives. There are, of course, entire books dedicated to cognitive therapy. Although these modules can certainly be used as a stand-alone guide, they are not meant to provide a comprehensive discussion of cognitive therapy. The reader is referred to other sources for more thorough descriptions of cognitive therapy with children and adolescents (Friedberg, McClure, & Garcia, 2009; Kendall, 2006; Reinecke, Dattilio, & Freeman, 2003).

This is the first of two emotion regulation modules focused on cognitive skills. The skills presented in this module are general and basic; Module 8 presents cognitive strategies related to specific emotions, describing ways to help kids think about thoughts related to sadness, fear, worry, and anger.

WHEN TO USE THIS MODULE

This module is designed for use when a major contributor to a client's difficulties involves patterns of thinking that interfere with optimal emotion regulation. Or, to borrow a phrase from a client, this module is designed for clients with "stinking thinking" when it comes to emotion.

Cognitive skills are an arguably more advanced set of skills than those covered in earlier modules. *Advanced* here means the client will already need to possess some basic emotion skills. For example, a client who understands that her actions can influence her emotions probably has enough background to successfully complete this module.

The intention here is not to make the module seem too difficult for most clients. In fact, cognitive strategies are commonly found in treatment programs for a variety of problems, and studies using the approaches often include rather young children in their samples. However, as noted above, cognitive strategies are more sophisticated than the strategies covered in previous modules, particularly when considering them as methods of emotion regulation. As a result, therapists may find it useful to proceed through the earlier modules before arriving here, because there is a progression. On the other hand, though, some clients may already have a good grasp on the content covered in the earlier modules, so starting with this module is certainly an option.

OBJECTIVES

The goal is to help clients understand that: (1) thoughts, feelings, and behaviors are related to each other; (2) different thoughts have different impacts on feelings and behaviors; (3) there are particular sorts of thoughts people have that make them feel better or worse; and (4) there are ways to help people think about and change their thoughts to help them feel better.

PROCEDURES

Step 1. Regulating Emotion: An Introduction

If Step 1 from Module 4 has not already been covered with the client, the therapist can use material from it as an introduction to the utility of emotion regulation. If therapists have already covered the material, though, there is no need to repeat it unless the client could benefit from the review.

Step 2. Using Thoughts to Deal with Feelings

Overview

The second step is divided into four subsections, each representing an important conceptual point to teach and practice with clients: (1) the cognitive triangle (also known as the triangle of thinking, feeling, and doing), (2) identifying thoughts, (3) diagnosing thoughts, and (4) changing thoughts.

Teach

*How You Think Influences What You Do and How You Feel; If You Change
Your Thinking, Your Feelings May Change Too*

The Cognitive Triangle. The triangle of thoughts–feelings–behaviors (see Figure 1), sometimes referred to as the cognitive triangle, can be a useful tool for helping clients visualize the relationship between the way they think, feel, and act. Most readers will be familiar with the triangle, so the description here will be brief.

The beauty of the triangle is its simplicity; many clients will be able to explain it without much prompting. For example, if you have a thought like, "I think I won't be very good at drawing," then that thought will increase feelings of anxiety about drawing, perhaps leading to the choice to avoid drawing. Similarly, though, a thought like "I know how to draw a pretty good funny face" might make you feel less anxious and more amused, perhaps leading you to want to draw.

Here is a case example in which the therapist blends in the triangle to help this client, Chelsea, a 16-year-old whose primary problems include depression and disruptive behaviors, including occasional suspensions from school. Here, the conversation is focused on Chelsea's efforts to deal with a peer who regularly tries to bother her (recently, for example, by implying that Chelsea's boyfriend is cheating on her).

THERAPIST: So, let's think about that triangle we talk about so much.

CHELSEA: Yeah—the magic triangle.

THERAPIST: So, Tameka came up to you and then . . . Let's use the triangle to see how this situation went.

CHELSEA: Yeah, so I was minding my own business. And then she just comes up and gets all up in my face and I was like . . .

THERAPIST: Okay, whoa. Let's play it back real slow. So you see Tameka coming. So what happened before she got there? Look at the triangle. What happened with these three things?

CHELSEA: Okay, well, hmm. I guess I had a thought, like, "Here comes that b-*&%^ again."

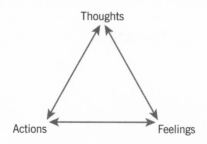

FIGURE 1. The cognitive triangle.

THERAPIST: And what impact did that thought have on your feelings or actions?

CHELSEA: Well, that got me ready to fight, I was mad.

THERAPIST: Ready for action—and a feeling! So did anything happen next, in the triangle? Like, did your feeling angry lead to other thoughts?

CHELSEA: Maybe. I looked at her and tried to see what she might be thinking. Is that a thought? I mean, I thought, "She is coming to cause some trouble."

THERAPIST: Right! You're getting good at this. That's a good example of how the triangle works.

Identifying Thoughts. With the triangle in hand, the next general step in cognitive work is what can be thought of as "mining for thoughts." Some clients will be reluctant to admit that they have many thoughts, using the infamous refrains of "I don't know" or "Nothing" in response to questions like, "What thoughts were you having?" or "What were you thinking?" In the "Practice: Activities and Games" section, any of the games can be adapted to help with this understanding. Although each of the games is designed to work on thoughts of hypothetical others, therapists are encouraged to adapt them to work directly with situations (and thoughts) pertinent to the client. In the end, the point of this step is simply to help clients learn that everyone has thoughts most of the time. The goal at this point is not to evaluate or change those thoughts, but to learn to enumerate them.

Diagnosing Thoughts. Once a client can identify thoughts and generate different thoughts for the same situation, a next step is to turn a discerning (scientific, not harsh or judgmental) eye toward the thoughts. Two important goals of this discernment (or examination of thoughts) are to notice patterns of the client's thinking and increase awareness of which thoughts are important to the client. Many readers are likely familiar with the *core belief* work initially promoted by Aaron Beck and Albert Ellis, among others.

One way to teach this is to create a list of thinking traps into which all people fall. Knowing about those traps makes them easier to avoid in the future. The following are some common thinking traps.

All-or-nothing thinking: Thinking of outcomes or situations in absolute versus relative terms. Examples: "I will never do well at math." "I always mess up in soccer."

Arbitrary inference: That is, jumping the gun, like when someone draws a conclusion quickly and on the basis of limited evidence. Examples: "That person did not smile at me. He hates me." "I got the first answer wrong on the test. I will fail."

Catastrophization: That is, making a mountain out of a molehill, as when someone assumes that an outcome will be magnificently bad, often out of all proportion to the situation. Example: "My friend is mad at me. I will never have another friend again." "I think I did badly on the history final. I will fail and my parents will ground me for life."

Emotional reasoning: When someone assumes that what he feels is true, and a fact, instead of evaluating all of the other facts available. Example: "I feel like I will never get good at the piano. It must be true."

Hostile attribution bias: When someone assumes that others' intentions are hostile, even in situations where it is hard to read the other person's intentions. Example: "That person bumped into me. He meant to hurt me."

Mind reading: When someone assumes that she can read others' minds and/or intentions. Examples: "My boyfriend hasn't called me today. He is angry with me for some reason." "My teacher is looking at me funny. She thinks I am an idiot."

Overgeneralization: When someone takes one negative event and assumes that it has meaning that pervades his whole life. Example: "I missed that shot. I am never going to make another shot."

Overpersonalization: When someone assumes that a situation is necessarily occurring because of her or that the situation is in relation to her. Example: "My mom seems mad today. It must be because of something I did."

Selective abstraction: That is, looking for the bad news, like when someone focuses only on some of the available evidence in order to draw a conclusion. Example: "My teacher mentioned that my report needed some edits. He hated it."

The goal with this step is *not* to convince clients that these traps are to be avoided. Instead, as it is with the whole of cognitive work, the goal is to help clients see that these traps exist, to help them understand how the traps affect feelings and behaviors, and to encourage clients to experiment with new and different ways of thinking.

Several of the activities and games listed in the "Practice: Activities and Games" section can be used to demonstrate how these thinking traps work, especially the What's Your Guess? Game.

Evaluating and Changing Thoughts. Sometimes people can change the way they think to help themselves handle feelings more effectively. They often do so by changing the way they are thinking so that their thoughts are more in line with the "reality" of the situation and/or more conducive to coping effectively.

The hardest part of using cognitive strategies as emotion regulation is guiding clients from *noticing they have thoughts that are less than helpful* to *doing something about it*. As will be detailed shortly, this fourth teaching point is fraught with much potential peril, and some recent approaches to cognitive work even suggest that it may not be necessary—that simple observation and acceptance of thoughts may be sufficient in some instances. Whereas there may be some utility to an "observe and accept" approach, there are often times when a client's thinking has gotten *stuck*. For such cases, identifying alternative, coping thoughts may be an important skill.

Before getting to the ways of practicing, however, it seems prudent to review some potential concerns and/or misunderstandings that some readers may have about cognitive strategies.

Myths about Cognitive Therapy Approaches. A few autobiographical comments may be helpful here as a preface. I have spent more than a dozen years now training therapists who come from a variety of backgrounds on how to do cognitive therapy. Many of the folks I have trained have had quite limited experiences with cognitive therapy and CBT, and some even have a background in disliking it! As a result, I have encountered many reservations and (mis)understandings about using cognitive strategies with clients. This brief section will list and discuss some common misconceptions about how cognitive strategies works.

Full disclosure: at the outset, it is worth noting that some of the misconceptions are even held by those in the scientific community, and it is likely that some cognitive therapy as provided is similar to the therapy depicted in the myths listed below. Nevertheless, what follows is a guide to what *not* to do.

Myth 1: The Goal Is to Convince My Client to Think More Rationally. This is an incorrect and potentially quite damaging misconception. Many times when training folks in cognitive strategies, I observe therapists role-playing what they think cognitive strategies look like. This often happens after several hours of other successful role plays, during which therapists have demonstrated how skilled they are in managing the client–therapist relationship and presenting new material in a supportive manner. Sometimes, though, once they are asked to role-play cognitive strategies, therapists can become incredibly prescriptive. Instead of exploring and collaborating with a client, they become either bossy or reassuring. As one example, here is an exchange between a therapist and client when discussing an upcoming social challenge—having to ask for help in a store:

THERAPIST: So how can you find out where the game is that you want?

ALYSIA: Well, I guess I could just look around the store.

THERAPIST: And if you cannot find it?

ALYSIA: Ask someone for help?

THERAPIST: How would that work? What would happen?

ALYSIA: Well, I don't know. They might think I was stupid for not knowing.

THERAPIST: Maybe. But remember, the employees are there to help you find things. And you are not supposed to know where things are in their store.

The therapist here is not particularly bossy, but she does all of the cognitive work for the client. Many times, such an approach can "feel" quite helpful, yet it may effectively shut down the discussion and reduce the chance for learning to occur. This is the age-old problem of giving the client a fish but not teaching her *how* to fish. In this case, it is plausible that the client does not even want the assistance the therapist offers her. Rather than providing an opportunity for Alysia to learn about her own thinking, the therapist simply gives her some different ways to think about the situation (one overall goal) without helping her understand how she would get there on her own.

Next is a re-do of the same scenario, taking a different approach.

THERAPIST: So how can you find out where the game is that you want?

ALYSIA: Well, I guess I could just look around the store.

THERAPIST: And if you cannot find it?

ALYSIA: Ask someone for help?

THERAPIST: How would that work? What would happen?

ALYSIA: Well, I don't know. They might think I was stupid for not knowing.

THERAPIST: Sounds like you have a guess about what the person might think about you—that she would think you were stupid. Remember the triangle we talked about, with thoughts, feelings, and actions?

ALYSIA: Um, yeah.

THERAPIST: I wonder what the thought "She will think I am stupid" will do to the feelings and actions.

ALYSIA: Well, it won't feel good.

THERAPIST: Probably not. When I think someone is thinking I am stupid, I feel crummy. Let's think this through together. Imagine you work in a store for a minute. Like Target.

ALYSIA: Like I am an employee there?

THERAPIST: Yeah, exactly. Now imagine I come up and ask you where I can find the toasters. What do you think about me?

ALYSIA: Because you asked me about toasters? I work there, right? So I think I would just tell you where they are. I mean, it's my job.

THERAPIST: Interesting. You would just tell me. What would you think of me for asking where the toasters were?

> ALYSIA: Nothing, really. I mean, why would I think something about you? You just want a toaster.
>
> THERAPIST: Right. Good. So if you worked at Target and a customer did not know where something was in the store, you would think, "I will tell that person."

The bottom line here is that the goal when doing cognitive work with clients is *not* to convince them to think a particular way. Instead, help them practice a way of thinking about and evaluating their thoughts (particularly, for the purposes of this book, in relation to how those thoughts affect their feelings).

Myth 2: Reassuring Clients Is a Good Way to Help Them Feel Better. This is a corollary to the first misconception and may stem from the experience some therapists have working with clients who have thoughts that are not just obviously making things worse but that are absolutely counter to the reality. In such cases, many therapists can be sorely tempted to offer reassurance. The case example that follows demonstrates how this can look.

> THERAPIST: So for homework, you are going to practice talking to your foster mom twice this week about something that upsets you that happens at school or with friends.
>
> PATTY: I don't know. She won't have time for that.
>
> THERAPIST: Sure she will. We talked about that with her.
>
> PATTY: But she seems busy and irritated when I try to talk to her. She doesn't really want to hear about that stuff anyway.
>
> THERAPIST: Sure she does. I know you are feeling concerned that she won't have time, but she and I talked, and I think she will be glad to hear about this.
>
> PATTY: I don't know.

Here, again, the therapist does the cognitive work for the client, preventing the client from learning how to do that work herself. This example may seem obvious, but a similar scenario can play out more subtly in many sessions. In a sense, almost any time a client has a thought (or guess) about some situation, helping her examine the thought can be a fruitful way to reinforce the lessons of cognitive therapy. Instead of reassuring, therapists can use a client's doubts and concerns as a means to explore and gather evidence, thereby practicing these valuable cognitive skills. So as with the previous example, here is a "take two."

> THERAPIST: So for homework, you are going to practice talking to your foster mom twice this week about something that upsets you that happens at school or with friends.
>
> PATTY: I don't know. She won't have time for that.
>
> THERAPIST: Hmm, sounds like you have a guess about how this is going to go.
>
> PATTY: I don't think it will go too well.

THERAPIST: What do you think will happen?

PATTY: I don't know. She won't listen or she will be annoyed.

THERAPIST: Okay, that sounds like two or three guesses right there. One, she won't have time. Two, she won't listen. And three, she will be annoyed. Remember the triangle *(points to the cognitive triangle on the wall)*?

PATTY: Oh, yeah.

THERAPIST: Why am I pointing to it now?

PATTY: I am having thoughts and those are making me feel like I don't want to do this.

THERAPIST: Right—good memory! So what can we do when we have thoughts that upset us?

PATTY: Look at them.

THERAPIST: Excellent—look at them. To use a fancy science-y phrase, we can gather evidence to test out whether thoughts are good guesses or not-so-good guesses. Let's think together about the three guesses you have about how this homework is going to go.

In this example, the therapist has to do a lot more work in the sense that she has to take more time and she still has not gotten to the point of assessing the thoughts. As is hopefully becoming clear, though, the goals here are *process* oriented and not *outcome* oriented. By taking the extra time, one can teach a method to clients—one that they can generalize and use in multiple situations—instead of feeding them platitudes like "think positive" and "it will go better than you think."

Myth 3: Cognitive Therapy Is about Teaching Kids to Think Positive. Teaching clients to think happy thoughts is *not* the goal of cognitive work. As described earlier, the goal is to teach and practice a different way of relating to thoughts that involves critically evaluating the thoughts in relation to how they help or hinder what the client wants to accomplish. This is a subtle point and one that is easily lost on many clients. As hard as I try on this particular point when doing cognitive work, I still hear my clients tell me late in therapy, "I just thought positively about it and it turned out all right." I have learned to live with that misunderstanding because some clients will have trouble developmentally understanding the subtle notion of evaluating thoughts, and it is possible that positive thinking really is the way to go sometimes. In general, though, it is best to persevere in teaching clients what may be a different way of thinking about their thoughts.

Why Does the Problem of Overly Prescriptive Cognitive Work Occur? First, there are stereotypes about cognitive work that create a straw man out of the approach—a *thought fixer* who prescribes the *right way* of thinking. So when people try to do cognitive work, some feel that their job is to "fix" thoughts. The caricature of cognitive work has been perhaps strengthened by caricatures of how some early cognitive therapists did their work (particularly Albert Ellis) and by some of the terms (*thinking errors* or *distortions*) that are used in describing cognitive therapy.

Second, the cognitive approach is a structured one. Therapists who are less familiar with structured approaches may find themselves feeling anxious about trying something new, overemphasizing structure to the point of rigidity, and taking an overly prescriptive and explanatory stance in sessions.

A third and final reason that may lead to the overly prescriptive approach is that cognitive work is deceptively challenging. Cognitive work appears so easy at first—the "errors" in others' thoughts are sometimes so glaring. Can it really be so simple as pointing them out and offering a few alternatives? However, helping a client learn the broad method of *how to think about thoughts* is difficult and painstaking. One must go slow and be patient, particularly with child and adolescent clients. Even when one understands the need to avoid the tendency to do the work for the clients and the temptation to reassure clients when they think negatively, one can easily find oneself falling into that trap.

So before transitioning to a few approaches to teaching cognitive strategies of emotion regulation to clients, here is some preliminary advice on avoiding the trap of overly prescriptive cognitive work.

Be Captain of the Impartiality Squad. The therapist's role is to remain impartial about a client's thoughts. She is not to judge the thoughts, declaring some "good" or "positive" and others "negative" or "errors." Instead, the therapist takes the role of a coinvestigator (with the client) in examining the thoughts the client is having and considering the impact of thinking in different ways about the situation. Some therapists have even commented at first that they worry they are being a little mean when acting as the captain of the impartiality squad. Some clients may want therapists to tell them what to do or think. But as tempting as it will be to nudge clients toward more adaptive thinking and away from the thoughts that most distress them, the goal instead is to engage in an analytic process with each thought and consider how it helps and/or hinders the client's goals.

As a result, a particularly hard part of the job is to avoid the impression that one has a stake in a particular thought or kind of thought. The simple truth here is that it is really hard to know which thoughts will help. Context can be a critical determinant. What helps at one time or in one place may be less helpful at another time or in another place.

Teach Fishing. Remember the adage, "Give a person a fish, you feed him for a day. Teach him to fish and you feed him for a lifetime." Offering reassurance comes naturally to many mental health workers, but remember that the goal is to model a way of approaching thoughts so that clients are prepared to handle the thoughts they have now as well as the thoughts that will come down the river later. Questions that are often useful in this work include:

- "What is the evidence for and against the thought?"
- "What would the consequences be of believing and/or acting on the thought?"
- "What other thoughts are there?"
- "What thoughts will help you act or feel in a way consistent with your goals?"

How Do Therapists Like the Taste of Their Own Medicine? A third idea that may help therapists struggling with how to teach cognitive strategies is to turn the tables: imagine yourself as the client and recall when people have tried to do cognitive work with you. How useful has it been to have people tell you things like:

- "Don't worry about that—it's no big deal."
- "She wasn't saying anything bad about you; she's just been in a bad mood lately."
- "Don't get bent out of shape about that. He didn't know you cared so much about it."

It is true that sometimes these reassurances can be helpful and supportive. But there are plenty of times when this advice pushes you into a disagreement with the advice giver, thereby strengthening your belief. What started off as a casual thought becomes a hardening position.

Similarly, unqualified validation of a person's thinking can also be problematic. Consider these thoughts:

- "That really is a big deal."
- "She can be really mean sometimes."
- "You are right to be mad. He was being a real jerk."

Again, the support is sometimes appreciated, but simply agreeing with the person may not help him get unstuck.

Now, none of this is to say that one should change how one acts as a *friend*. As friends, sometimes we disagree and other times we provide support, acceptance, and agreement. Furthermore, therapists may sometimes serve a similar supportive role. However, when doing cognitive work, these two tactics should generally be avoided in favor of the challenging middle path: looking hard at thoughts without judging them.

How to Teach Cognitive Strategies. With that considerable, and largely prefatory, material already discussed, it is time to transition to four common methods for teaching cognitive work: (1) remember Socrates, (2) be a scientist/detective, (3) follow the downward arrow, and (4) foster "other thought" generation.

Remember Socrates. What is the Socratic method? As most readers will recall, Socrates taught in a way that involved asking questions, instead of providing answers, as a way to encourage critical thinking. The method has evolved for use as a pedagogical and therapeutic tool. The method generally involves asking questions that are open ended and exploratory. Relevant to cognitive therapy, there are several categories of question one may ask in using the Socratic method. These include the following.

Clarification questions. With these questions, the aim is to gather more information. Such questions include: "What do you mean by *X*?" "What are your ideas about how to handle that?"

Reason/evidence questions. These questions represent a common approach in cognitive work because the overall goal is to teach clients to evaluate thoughts. Evidence is one way to evaluate them, and so asking questions about evidence is a critical way to teach and practice. Such questions include: "What evidence do you have that that is true?" "What are your reasons for saying that?" "What would convince you that you are correct (or incorrect) about that?"

Point-of-view questions. These questions allow the client (and therapist) to consider another person's viewpoint. Here one asks questions that require the client to think of how others might perceive the situation. Examples of this sort of question include: "What would someone who disagrees with you say?" "What would someone who wants to help you feel more (or less) upset about this say?"

Implication/consequence questions. As the name implies, these questions involve asking the client to imagine the consequences or implications of their thoughts. These sorts of questions can take at least three different tacks. The first involves directing clients to imagine the "worst-case scenario" and is related to the *downward-arrow* principle that will be discussed shortly. Examples of the downward-arrow style questions would include: "What would happen if that thought turns out to be true?" "What would be the worst thing that could happen?"

The second approach is akin to asking the client to examine evidence, albeit hypothetical evidence, with questions like this: "What is the likelihood of that occurring—and how do you know that?" "What are some alternative things that could happen?"

A third approach of these "implications" questions is what I sometimes call the "Dr. Phil" method, after TV host and psychologist Dr. Phil McGraw. Please note that the recommendation here is not to use the judgmental tone that Dr. Phil sometimes takes, but rather to borrow the spirit of the questions. Examples include: "How has thinking like that worked for you?" "How would we know if that way of thinking was working?"

Although effective, being Socratic when teaching cognitive strategies is time consuming. However, persistence with the Socratic method improves the client's likelihood of retaining the message that examining one's thinking can help one deal with complicated feelings.

Cognitive Therapy as Scientific or Detective Work. Recall the notion of the therapist as co-investigator. Imagine that the client and therapist are engaged in a scientific study designed to learn more about the client's thoughts and how those thoughts have an impact on his feelings. Alternatively, one might consider the therapist's role as that of a codetective who is gathering clues or evidence to see which theory about a crime is true. Or imagine that therapist and client play the roles of prosecuting and defense attorneys. In any of these metaphors, the important process of cognitive therapy is that of gathering and evaluating evidence, with the goal being to see whether there is good reason to change the way one is thinking. The case example here exemplifies one way of doing this.

THERAPIST: Let's think about this like we're detectives. Do you know any detectives from books or TV?

KALEY: Well, I've read a few old Nancy Drew books my mom had around. She's like a detective, right?

THERAPIST: Right—good one. Nancy Drew. What do detectives do?

KALEY: Well, they try to figure out who did a crime, like a murder.

THERAPIST: Yep. And how do they figure it out?

KALEY: Um, I don't know. I guess they get some clues and put them together?

THERAPIST: That's right. They get clues, like evidence, right. They look for the evidence— why?

KALEY: To see who did it.

THERAPIST: Right. How will they know?

KALEY: Well, the evidence will show them.

THERAPIST: Does all the evidence always point to the same answer?

KALEY: Um, I dunno.

THERAPIST: Let me ask that in different way. Imagine one clue was that that the person who did the crime was wearing jeans. Would that clue narrow the field down to one person? Is there only one person who was wearing jeans?

KALEY: Well, no. I mean, lots of people wear jeans.

THERAPIST: Yeah, they do. So just because the person wore jeans doesn't mean we know who did it yet. There is a lot of evidence to sort through. Detectives have to wait to see how all the evidence fits together. I have a game called Thought Detectives [described in the Practice section of this module] that is played a lot like how detectives work, except instead of investigating crimes, we are investigating thoughts.

The therapist may choose to liken this process to scientific thinking rather than detective work. In this metaphor, thoughts are guesses or hypotheses. To test hypotheses, clients gather evidence and then weigh that evidence. A bonus of the science metaphor is that to test hypotheses, one often needs to conduct experiments, and those experiments can be actual tasks that clients do in therapy to test the thoughts/guesses. For example, if a client thinks that he will be terrible at playing soccer, the therapist could work with him to define what *terrible* means (i.e., how one would measure terrible) and design multiple tests of his soccer prowess and then measure his performance.

Follow the Downward Arrow. Another important tenet in using cognitive techniques with clients is concerned with what is called the *downward arrow*. Sometimes, the first thoughts identified by the client may appear rather superficial. The downward arrow involves following one thought through to its *worst-case* scenario. The notion here is that although the first thought or two that come to mind may not seem particularly distressing, digging deeper may lead to more distressing thoughts that can help shed light on a client's emotional predicament. "Digging deeper" does not necessarily mean delving deeply in a client's history; instead, the deep digging should root out the ramifications or *meaning* of a particular thought.

In practice, the downward arrow involves asking a series of questions that lead the client from an initial thought to its worst possible conclusion or meaning. Questions might include:

- "What would happen then or next?"
- "What would it mean if that happened?"
- "Imagine the worst happened—then what?"

The goal with downward arrow is to find the *bottom* of a client's thinking; that is, what terrible or unpleasant outcome most worries, saddens, or angers the client. Although it is often the case that finding the bottom is simply a matter of asking questions, sometimes a therapist will need to suggest possible negative outcomes, as not all clients are aware of the thoughts or predictions that most distress them until they hear them. It is worth mentioning, too, that there are individual differences as to what is at the *bottom* of the arrow. The following clinical excerpt provides an example of the process recommended.

THERAPIST: One thought you have in that situation is you won't do well on the test?
ZEKE: Yeah, I guess.

THERAPIST: Okay, so let's say that you didn't do well on the test. What would happen then?

ZEKE: Um, like I did really bad?

THERAPIST: How bad would be the worst you can imagine?

ZEKE: Well, like what if I failed?

THERAPIST: Okay. Let's say you failed. Then what would happen?

ZEKE: I don't know.

THERAPIST: What would your guess be? The worst thing that would happen next?

ZEKE: The worst? Well, I could fail the class?

THERAPIST: Okay, you failed the class. And then what?

ZEKE: And then maybe I would fail 10th grade?

THERAPIST: Let's say that happened? Then what?

ZEKE: Mom and stepdad would freak out—they'd be super mad.

THERAPIST: Let's say they got really mad. Then what?

The therapist here continued on for another minute or so, getting down to the notion that his mother and stepfather would end up being right that he (Zeke) would never amount to anything in his life and would be a loser, just like his biological father. In the end, a major concern for Zeke was ending up like his biological father, who had been unemployed for years (despite the perception of many that he was capable of doing more) and who had been a no-show for much of Zeke's childhood. Knowing about these concerns greatly helped the therapist to tailor cognitive work moving forward.

And as discerning readers may note, the path to this outcome is not obvious from the first thought. In some cases, a concern about failing a test may lead to fears about one's academic future or concerns that family will stop loving you. The downward arrow helps you get to these deep concerns.

Foster "Other Thought" Generation. Up until this point, the focus of the strategies has been thought identification and refinement. In a sense, a significant portion of cognitive work is assessment-related, and there are risks to moving too quickly into anything more than identification of thoughts. Indeed, as has been a theme in the module, thinking about cognitive work as a way to *fix* thoughts is plain wrong. However, cognitive work is certainly not simply a matter of helping clients identify their thoughts; another important component is generating alternative thoughts. Specifically, the goal is to help clients become better at generating thoughts that will (ideally) be more helpful to them. Just how does one do this, though?

There are myriad ways. Two are already described: using Socratic questions and engaging in detective work or scientific thinking. These strategies are good ones because they are less directive, require work from the client, and generally end up with ideas that are well fitted to the client. However, there are times when either these strategies do not work or more direct suggestive work is needed from the therapist. Below are two additional strategies a therapist can use when he believes he needs to provide specific alternative thought suggestions.

1. **Brainstorm other thoughts.** The therapist can work with the client to create a list of other thoughts that a person might have in a given situation. Like any brainstorm, the idea is to generate a number of possibilities and then consider their benefits and downsides. It often helps to be clear that, at first, the goal is simply to list out as many thoughts as possible without evaluating them. Then, when it's time to weight their pros and cons, referencing the cognitive triangle can be a helpful (e.g., "If you had the thought 'The punishment will be a bummer but it will be over in a few minutes,' what would happen to your feelings?").

2. **Explain the rationale behind helpful/counter/coping thoughts.** In contrast to the indirect route of Socratic questions and the meandering route of detective work, it can sometimes be useful to be quite direct about the goal of generating thoughts that will help clients cope. Although many children are reluctantly in therapy, some are more eager for change. If a client understands and agrees that one goal of therapy is to identify helpful thoughts (or counter or coping thoughts), the going can become a bit easier.

Practice: Activities and Games

What follows are three activities and games designed to help clients practice marking connections between feelings and thoughts.

Cognitive Shuttle

This game is designed to establish the basics of cognitive work—that people have thoughts and those thoughts influence our feelings and actions. The game combines physical activity and a matching task; as a result, it can be particularly useful when working with younger and/or active clients. The game as presented here has a number of possible variations. Therapists should feel free to adapt and/or modify these ideas to their own and their clients' preferences.

Preparation. Therapists will need a set of signs that categorize thoughts and a set of cards that each list a situation and one emotion-related thought. A description of these two components follows.

Signs. The signs are used to categorize thoughts. Given the variability in development among clients, three possible sign sets are described:

1. **Simple signs.** For young clients or those challenged by complex concepts, three signs may suffice: (a) "Helpful thought," (b) "Unhelpful thought," and (c) "Neutral thought."
2. **Direction + feelings signs.** A more advanced set of signs can reflect a thought's impact on particular emotions (e.g., more worried, less angry). This requires multiple feelings signs (e.g., happy, sad, afraid) as well as a PLUS sign and a MINUS sign. The player touches a feeling sign and the PLUS sign (meaning an increase in the feeling) or MINUS sign (meaning a decrease in the feeling). Of course, some thoughts can influence more than one feeling, so clients can touch more than one feeling.
3. **Thought category signs.** An alternative and even more advanced set of signs can contain thought categories, such as: (a) overgeneralization, (b) catastrophization, (c) overestimation, and (d) selective abstraction. Here, the client would touch the pattern or patterns reflected in each thought. It can be useful when using this approach to review the definitions of these thought patterns (even consider writing a summary on the sign) and/or create a picture that represents the category, like a magnifying glass for selective abstraction (i.e., looking carefully at one thing). For more helpful thoughts, the client can identify which pattern is countered by the thought.

Situation and Thought (S&T) Cards. Therapists may opt to prepare these S&T cards in advance of playing, although the cards can easily be made as part of the meeting with the client, with the client contributing to their creation. What is needed are a variety of different emotional situations, each associated with several different thoughts. It is usually easiest to generate a set of situations and then use those situations to generate the thoughts.

Here are a few goals to keep in mind while making the S&T cards. First, aim for several *less-than-helpful* thoughts. Although having a list of helpful, coping thoughts has its benefits, it is important to get the *less helpful* thoughts out on the table and consider them carefully. Second, try to include some thoughts relevant to the client's own situation. Third, strive for a variety of situations that will lead to different sorts of feelings.

Several examples of possible S&T cards are below:

Situation: The teacher has just called on you.

Thoughts:
　　"Oh no! I'm going to get the answer wrong!"
　　"Am I in trouble?"
　　"What was she just saying?"
　　"I'm so glad I did the homework last night."
　　"She always picks me."

Situation: Some kids are looking at you in the lunchroom.

Thoughts:
"I'm wearing a cool outfit."
"I must have something weird on my back."
"They are making fun of me."
"They want to beat me up."

Situation: You've called your friend three times and she hasn't called you back.

Thoughts:
"She hates me now."
"She must have gotten busted by her parents again."
"She's spending time with her other friends and not me."
"Maybe she's hurt!"

Situation: A kid bumps into you at the mall.

Thoughts:
"He seems pretty clumsy."
"What's his problem? He did that on purpose."
"It's a little crowded here."
"I'm such a clumsy loser!"

Situation: Your dad is late picking you up from a friend's house.

Thoughts:
"Car accident!"
"He got lost again."
"He got too busy at work to come get me."
"He forgot."

Situation: You forgot to do your homework.

Thoughts:
"No biggie! I can get it done before class."
"I am going to get called on for sure."
"I'll probably fail the class now."
"I'm an idiot!"

Gameplay. The signs are placed in various locations so that the player has to move to touch each one. That is, the signs should be far enough apart from each other to require movement between them. The deck of S&T cards is placed face down on the table. A player draws a card and reads the situation and then chooses one (any) thought from the list and reads that as well. The player then runs over to the sign that she thinks is most appropriate for the thought, tags it, and then runs back to where she started. The therapist can clarify and/or gently correct the client if the choice is clearly incorrect. After the first "shuttle," the player reads the next thought on the card and runs to the appropriate sign for that thought.

Optional Add-On. After all thoughts on the card have been categorized, the client and therapist can choose to add one or more other thoughts to the card. The goal of this add-on activity is *not* to emphasize the "goodness" of the new thoughts (recall the therapist's role as captain of the impartiality squad), but instead simply to generate alternative thoughts and evaluate the impact of those thoughts on feelings. Although it is generally best to encourage the client to produce the new thoughts, it can sometimes be helpful for therapists "to get the party started," especially early on, when a client may not have a deep well to go to for these thoughts. As these new alternative thoughts are generated, the client can run and touch the appropriate signs.

Alternate Version 1: Cognitive Targets. This game is similar to Cognitive Shuttle but has a simpler set-up. The same signs can be used, but the cards should include only situations (thoughts on the S&T cards could be covered up with Post-its). Players take turns as follows: (1) Player 1 selects a situation card; (2) Player 2 chooses one of the signs by tossing a *missile* (crumpled-up paper works fine—choose something safe!) at the sign; and (3) Player 1 must generate a thought for the situation on the card consistent with whatever sign Player 2 targeted. Play can be repeated multiple times for each situation.

Alternate Version 2: Cognitive Hoops. This game is exactly the same as Cognitive Targets, except labeled cups or containers are used instead of signs. A "ball" (crumpled paper works fine, a Ping-Pong ball is also good) is thrown at the cups.

Alternate Version 3: Cognitive Feats of Strength. With a title inspired by an episode of the 1990s television show *Seinfeld*, this variant assigns a *feat of strength* to each sign. Rather than running to a sign to categorize the thought, as in Cognitive Shuttle, the player performs the feat of strength on the appropriate categorizing sign to indicate his selection. Gameplay involves a player drawing an S&T card, reading the situation, and then reading the thoughts one at a time. After each thought, the player performs the feat of strength associated with the correct category. Example feats of strength include might include: (1) standing on one foot for 30 seconds, (2) doing five wall pushups, (3) assuming a yoga position, or (4) doing five jumping jacks. The constraints of the setting will dictate the list of feats.

Thought Detectives

This is a game in which the therapist and client pose as detectives trying to solve a mystery in which clues are revealed one at a time. The game is akin to the popular murder mystery dinner party games that are sold in book and game stores. The mysteries here are not crimes, but instead are challenging and ambiguous situations that arise in children's lives.

Preparation. This game requires some preparation time, but if a therapist preps for a few of these, the materials can be reused with many clients. Doing the preparation in the meeting is also possible, although that does require quick thinking and/or a creatively oriented client.

Step 1. Choose a Stem. First, the therapist needs to construct at least one mystery to be solved. Three basic scenarios (stems) are provided here, but the possibilities are endless. Personalizing these to the therapist (and clientele) is worth the effort. A good rule of thumb is to have two or three prepared stems before going into a meeting to allow the client some choice and create the chance for a round 2 (or 3).

Scenario 1: The phone call mystery. A friend fails to call or text another character. Why hasn't he called back?

Scenario 2: The confusing teacher mystery. A teacher frowned at a student during class and asked to see that student after school. Why?

Scenario 3: The late pick-up mystery. A parent is late to pick up a child from an after-school activity. What happened?

Step 2. Create a Narrative. The goal is to create enough of a narrative so that there is mystery and ambiguity as well as some interest. Overly obvious situations will often fail to engage clients. Notice that in the example below, character names and ages are assigned. Designing the mysteries to feel personal makes the game more enjoyable and immersive for the client.

Scenario 1: The phone call mystery. Angelina and Cate have just become friends at Bellevue High School in the last few months. One Saturday morning, Cate calls Angelina but receives no callback for a few hours. She then sends a text message to Angelina. An hour later, Cate has received no reply. Why hasn't Angelina called or texted back?

Step 3: Generate Clues. The therapist generates a set of clues that she will reveal to the client one at a time. The clues should be listed individually on a sheet of paper or on separate index cards, and a good range is between three and seven clues (enough to generate some suspense, but not so many that the explanation becomes obvious). It is easiest to create clues for a mystery when those clues have an inherent order in which they should be revealed. In the example that follows, five clues are used.

Scenario 1: The phone call mystery. Clues presented in this order.

Clue 1. Cate saw Angelina talking to some of her other friends after school on Friday.

Clue 2. Angelina did not eat lunch with Cate on Friday.

Clue 3. Cate moved to Bellevue last year, but Angelina has lived here since she was in preschool.

Clue 4. Angelina's family is wealthier than Cate's.

Clue 5. Angelina left school early on Friday.

Gameplay. Anyone familiar with mystery dinner parties will quickly pick up on how this game is played. For those unfamiliar with such games, the game is played using the following steps.

1. Read through the narrative.
2. Draw the first clue and read it.
3. Using the clue as inspiration, generate possible solutions to the mystery. The therapist's work is to help the client see how the solutions are like guesses or thoughts the character in the story could have.
4. Discuss the consequences of each solution generated, using the cognitive triangle as the basis for discussion. In other words, how would the main character feel, and what would happen to her if she concluded that the solution to the mystery was the idea being discussed?
5. Have client state his best guess for the solution (and why). Write down the clue number and the guess.
6. Draw the next clue.
7. Repeat Steps 3, 4, and 5. Ensure that there is some discussion on how the new clue affected your thinking about the situation and how it supported (or not) the previously generated solution.
8. After the final clue is drawn, therapist and client should discuss (and, one hopes, agree on) what is the most likely solution given all the clues.
9. *Optional.* Reconsider each clue and discuss whether it would have made sense to guess the *final* solution when reading that clue.

What's Your Guess? Game

A colleague of mine, Bruce Chorpita, introduced me to the idea of referring to thoughts as *guesses*—a notion that inspired this game. The game is designed to help clients practice thought generation and examination, consistent with the teaching points of the module.

Preparation. The therapist should create a set of cards, each containing a few sentences describing a situation or a story. The stories should be incomplete, though. The characters in the story should be in the middle of something when the story "ends." To play a good round of the game, about seven cards are needed.

Two additional requirements for the stories on the cards: each one should have more than one person but fewer than five, and each story should have an important outcome pending, but almost no clues about what that outcome will be.

Here are a few example situations that could be used to start a deck of cards. The character listed in **bold** is the main character.

Scenario 1: Tom and **Sandy** worked on a class project together. The teacher is passing out the grades and approaches their table. Instead of handing them the graded papers, she asks to see **Sandy** in the hallway.

Scenario 2: Reginald sees his friend Tyler in the hall and waves to him. Tyler does not wave back.

Scenario 3: Grace and Cintia are playing. **Katie** comes over to them and asks if she can join them.

Scenario 4: Travis and **Abby** are in the after-school program at their school. **Abby's** mother is late picking her up today.

Gameplay. Someone shuffles the deck of cards and then Player 1 draws a card. Player 1 reads the card and offers a guess as to what the main character thinks will happen next. For Example 1 above, Player 1 might guess that Sandy will think that the teacher is going to punish her. Then Player 1 will then answer these questions:

- "*Why* would Sandy make that guess?"
- "*How* will Sandy feel if she makes that guess? What will she do?"
- "*What* if the first guess is wrong (i.e., the teacher is not going to punish Sandy)? What else might Sandy guess that would lead her to have a different feeling than she would have if she were punished?"

After the turn is complete, Player 2 can either (1) remain with the same card or (2) choose to draw a new one. If he chooses (1), then the task is to make a different guess than the first person.

Alternate Version 1: What about That Other Person? In this variation, guesses are offered for the other characters in the story. The same pattern of game-play applies.

Alternate Version 2: Escaping from a Trap. For this variation, a second set of cards is needed with the names of thinking traps on them (see the "Diagnosing Thoughts" section earlier in the module). At the start of the turn, a player draws both a Situation and a Trap card. The player then has two tasks. First, he must generate a thought for that situation consistent with the thinking trap. Next, he must generate a thought that would help him get out of the trap.

MODULE 8

Emotion Regulation Skills V
Emotion-Specific Cognitive Skills

This final module focuses on cognitive strategies related to specific emotions, describing ways to help kids evaluate thoughts related to sadness, fear, worry, and anger.

WHEN TO USE THIS MODULE

This module is designed for use when a major contributor to a client's difficulties is a lack of skill regulating one of four specific emotions: anger, worry, sadness, and fear. Specifically, the module addresses how a client's thinking patterns interfere with optimal emotion regulation. The same caveats offered at the start of Module 7 are relevant here. The strategies described do require a relatively mature client, one who can engage in some talk about his thoughts. It is also worth noting that although this module can be used without having already covered Module 7, the two do make a nice one-two combination.

OBJECTIVES

Objectives for this module are to teach and practice using cognitive emotion regulation skills related to the four specific feelings mentioned above: anger, worry, sadness, and fear.

PROCEDURES

Step 1. Emotion Regulation: An Introduction

If Step 1 from Module 4 has not already been covered with the client, the therapist can use material from it as an introduction to the utility of emotion regulation. If therapists have already covered the material, though, there is no need to repeat it unless the client could benefit from the review.

Step 2. Using Thoughts to Deal with Anger

Overview

Anger is a distressing and *activating* emotion, a feeling that by design inspires a person to circumvent thinking. As such, a main goal when using a cognitive emotion regulation approach with clients who struggle with anger is to increase the amount of time between when the emotion "starts" and when action begins: to *inhibit behavior* and *disinhibit thinking*. The basic approach to identifying and analyzing thoughts followed by generating other thoughts, described in Module 7, can be generally helpful. However, there are some specific cognitive interventions developed for anger that are worth considering, one of which is presented in some detail here: *perspective taking*.

Teach

How to Use Thoughts to Deal with Angry Feelings

Perspective Taking.   Perspective taking is a strategy discussed in Module 3 as a means to understand the feelings of another person. In this module, the strategy is simplified to provide the client with a method for slowing herself down when she's angry. There are three main points to make:

1. **There are many ways to see a situation.** A concrete way for the therapist to help the client understand this point is for the therapist and client to take up separate vantage points in a room and then each describe the things they can see and describe how those things look. Ideally, therapists can choose vantage points so that each person has a perspective that misses some things and distorts others.

2. **A situation can look different to different people.** It is important to extend this experience metaphorically to how some situations look different because of a person's internal experiences. In other words, two people may both see the same object and see it from the same place, but depending on who they each are and what they each have experienced, that object (or situation) can (and often does) have a different meaning. An easy way to do this is to tell a

story like the brief one introduced in Module 2 and repeated here: "Imagine a kid who was invited to eat ice cream. How would that client feel?" Many clients will respond that the child would feel excited and happy (and maybe hungry). Then ask the client to consider if he thinks the kid's feeling would be different if the kid was allergic to milk and the ice cream would actually make him sick. See the Omniscience (or Seeing All Sides) game in the "Practice: Activities and Games" section that follows to help practice this point.

3. **Different perspectives result in different feelings and behaviors.** This is a logical extension of the fact that people have different perspectives. The feelings and behaviors that arise from those perspectives can be quite different, even when those experiences are arguably the same.

Practice: Activities and Games

What follows are two brief ways to help clients practice experiencing anger and engaging in cognitive strategies to help regulate that anger.

Simulated Anger Memory Game

John Lochman and his colleagues at the University of Alabama describe a game that involves provoking client anger (safely) to allow the client to practice different ways of slowing down her anger response (see Larson & Lochman, 2011).[1]

In this game, the client is told that she will be playing a memory game in which she has to remember a set of cards. Cards are drawn and shown to the client one at a time for a brief time (a few seconds) and then each card is placed face down. Clients are asked to recall the card (or cards) shown. The therapist can start by showing one card at a time, asking for recall after each. Over time, the therapist can increase the number of cards shown before requesting the recall, making the memory task more demanding. What makes the game a challenge and related to emotion regulation is that as each card is shown, the therapist presents an emotional challenge. Examples of such challenges include: (1) the therapist annoying the client by calling her name in different voices; (2) the therapist (gently and with permission) teasing the client, calling her silly names; or (3) the therapist offering discouraging words (again with permission) during the activity (e.g., suggesting that the client will be unable to remember the cards). The idea here is to find a challenge that will irritate or anger the client enough so that she might be distracted from following through on the focal activity—in this case, remembering cards.

---

[1]Adapted from Larson and Lochman (2011). Copyright 2011 by The Guilford Press. Adapted by permission.

The therapist is encouraged before the game to help the client generate thoughts (and other strategies) to use during the "challenges" that will help her focus on remembering the cards. Thoughts might include:

"Stay focused."
"I can do this."
"That teasing is not true."
"What is on the card?"

Conducting this particular exercise requires great care on the part of the therapist, who should first make sure the client understands that this a game and that the therapist's teasing is pretend and not genuine. Second, the therapist should leave time to discuss the activity, with a focus on how the game affected the client's perceptions of her relationship with the therapist. Furthermore, the therapist should preface the game by saying that some clients have played this game and then worried that the therapist really did not like them or that the teasing was real, but that that was not the case. Despite all of the preparation, clients should have a chance to talk about any hurt feelings they might have after the game is over. Finally, although the game is an effective way to practice handling anger, it is not for all clients (nor all therapists); consider how the specific client would handle the game before attempting to play. Even with clients who will probably handle the game well, the therapist should proceed carefully.

Involving Siblings and Peers. Another way to help clients practice in simulated anger situations that does not involve the therapist being the anger provoker is to include siblings or peers (when possible). Same-age peers can be good helpers insofar as some clients will have trouble taking a therapist seriously in the role of a provocateur. The basic activity here is to role-play situations in which the client has trouble managing his anger. The client role-plays with a peer or sibling, with the peer/sibling playing the provocateur. The therapist plays the role of coach, working with the client before, during, and after role plays to come up with thoughts and other strategies to help manage the anger. The therapist can also vary the difficulty of the role play by working with the peer or sibling to increase or decrease the challenge level.

A clinical example may help to exemplify this approach. I once was supervising a therapist whose 11-year-old male client was getting into many fights because of his proclivity to respond to the slightest peer provocation as an invitation for a rumble. The therapist role-played teasing situations with the client, having even done some research to pick up some popular (language-appropriate) middle school insults. Despite the therapist's best efforts, the client laughed hysterically during the role plays, apparently finding her efforts at teasing hilarious. Although the client was able to practice what he might do and think differently in provocative situations, he was not getting any practice when he was actually upset. As a result, with the client's permission, the therapist involved his older brother in the role plays. The client was much less amused, and the practice became more heated and more valuable.

When involving siblings and/or peers, there are obviously a few rules: (1) one must get the client's permission; (2) one must prepare the sibling/peer for the role (this is not a time to assume good improvisational skills or the sibling or peer's understanding of the goals); and (3) one should have a good sense of whether the sibling/peer is trustworthy—not all siblings/peers are cut out to be helpful in this type of activity.

Omniscience (or Seeing All Sides)

This game helps clients practice the perspective-taking skill as one cognitive strategy to regulate anger.

Preparation. In advance of the game, therapists will need to prepare a set of scenarios written on index cards or sheets of paper. Ideally, some of the scenarios will be relevant to the client. Sample scenarios are listed here.

Scenario 1: Ty and Jack are in line for lunch. Ty gets his lunch tray full of food and heads for his seat. Jack bumps into Ty, upsetting his tray, and food spills everywhere.

Scenario 2: Francine and Helen are talking in the hallway at school. Their friend Wendy walks by in a hurry, laughing, with a new girl that Francine and Helen don't know. Francine says "Hi" to Wendy, but Wendy doesn't look at her.

Scenario 3: Brianna and Emily are friends in the same math class. One day the teacher returns their recent tests and Emily has scored much higher than Brianna.

Scenario 4: Kate and Garry's mother is late coming home from work again, so they have to stay with their grandmother, who can be strict. When their mother finally arrives at 6:30 P.M., Kate and Garry are hungry and their homework is not yet done.

Gameplay

1. Player 1 selects a scenario and reads it aloud.
2. Player 1 picks one of the characters in the scenario and tells or writes one perspective for that person. That is, the player is tasked with imagining

being the character and then listing one of the many different ways that the character might be thinking, feeling, and behaving in the situation. For the perspective offered, the player also describes what would happen next in the scenario. That is, the player considers the consequences of the character taking that perspective.

3. Once Player 1 is done, Player 2 adds another perspective.
4. Play goes back and forth between the players until no additional new perspectives can be offered related to the first character identified.
5. After the perspectives for the situation have been exhausted, the players agree on scoring, with 1 point awarded for each unique perspective.
6. Once scoring for the first character is established, Player 2 picks a different character from the scenario and the process starts anew.
7. The process is repeated until perspectives have been identified for each person in the scenario.
8. The game can end after one scenario or can be continued with additional scenarios.

Scoring. Note that, as mentioned in Step 5 of "Gameplay," players must agree on whether a perspective earns a point. A therapist's role, in addition to being an active player, is to help the client explain *why* the character would have a particular perspective and then helping the client consider the ramifications (good and bad) of each perspective he describes. If clients do not generate "negative" perspectives, the therapist should be sure to volunteer those. For example, in Scenario 2, the therapist could offer at least one of the following negative perspectives: (1) Wendy hates Francine, (2) Wendy was laughing at Francine, or (3) Helen knows why Wendy did not say "Hi" but won't say. In short, it is important to consider all sides, including those that are less positive or adaptive, since chances are the client is already taking some of those perspectives.

Step 3. Using Thoughts to Deal with Worries

Overview

What are worries but thoughts? Hence, it is probably not surprising that cognitive interventions are important for worry regulation. A trick here though is that because worry is all in the head, sometimes the goal is to get a client out of her head—not easy when the worrier views the worrying as functional. Many worriers will explain that if they did not worry so much, their problems would be worse. Indeed, it can sometimes be a challenge to define where problem solving and planning ahead end and where problematic worrying begins.

The basic cognitive strategies described in Module 7 can be useful for worriers, an observation that the published literature bears out insofar as worriers have strong outcomes when treated with programs containing cognitive interventions (e.g., Chorpita & Southam-Gerow, 2006). An additional concept, not described in Module 7, is *worry triage*.

Teach

Triage Those Worries

Worry triage involves separating out concerns (or worries) into at least three groups: (1) concerns that can be addressed directly and in short order (i.e., now); (2) concerns that can be addressed, but not immediately (i.e., later); and (3) concerns over which one has neither immediate nor later control (i.e., maybe never). The goal is to help worrying clients learn to sort through their worries and make these distinctions more accurately and quickly.

The overall method involves helping clients to see that they can exert some control over the worry process through a few avenues. First, clients can sort through and prioritize worries by considering (1) how pressing the worry is, (2) how solvable the worry is, and (3) how much agency the client has over the worry. Second, clients can be encouraged to weigh the costs and benefits of worrying about situations with some of the following characteristics: (1) the situation is one over which they have little or no control, (2) the situation is not a pressing one, and (3) the situation represents a remote and highly unlikely threat.

Such a conversation may be more successful if conducted using the Socratic method, with the therapist acting as captain of the impartiality squad (see Module 7 for details). Although the concept of worry triage is not captured in Module 7, many of the teaching points and games from that module can be useful when teaching clients to make distinctions among their worries.

Another important guideline described in Module 7 that bears repeating here: be wary of providing too many answers for clients. Therapists are urged to become aware of their tendencies to say things like, "Don't worry about that, it's no big deal." Instead, with worry triage, the therapist helps the client think through and sort his list of worries by asking questions like the following.

WORRY TRIAGE: SAMPLE QUESTIONS

1. What steps can I take to solve this problem?

2. What will happen if I stop thinking about this situation?

3. What will happen if I do nothing about this situation?

4. How soon will the negative outcomes I am worried about occur for this situation?

5. How would this situation rank in importance to solve, compared to others?

6. How much control do I have over this situation?

7. How would this situation rank in terms of how much control I have over it, compared to others?

8. How likely is the most negative outcome related to my worry if I do nothing except stop worrying about it?

9. How much less likely is that outcome if I do worry about it?

Practice: Activities and Games

Worry Sort

The object of the game is to sort the worries of a fictional set of characters.

Preparation. Two sets of cards are needed. The first, Character Cards, contain descriptions of a variety of youths. The second, Worry Cards, contain individual worries. It is best to have at least three Character Cards and at least 10 Worry Cards. Of course, some of the Worry Cards should be relevant to the client's worries, although it is also useful to include worries that are not particularly relevant to the client.

In addition to the Character and Worry Cards, the therapist should also prepare four signs: (1) "Worry Now," (2) "Worry Later," (3) "No Worry," and (4) "Not Sure."

Sample Character and Worry Cards are provided here.

CHARACTER CARDS

Character 1: Sal is a 12-year-old boy who goes to a public middle school. He lives with his mother and older sister. His dad lives in another town, and Sal doesn't get to see him much. Here are some of Sal's worries . . .

Character 2: Sally is a 15-year-old girl who goes to a small public high school. She lives with her mother and stepfather and her two half-siblings (a brother and sister), who are younger. She does well in school and wants to go to college. Here are some of Sally's worries . . .

WORRY CARDS

Worry 1: What if I fail algebra?

Worry 2: What if my mom or dad gets sick again?

Worry 3: What if mom or dad gets fired at work?

Worry 4. What if my social studies teacher yells at me tomorrow?

Worry 5. What if my friend Daniel moves to another school?

Worry 6. What if I get the swine flu?

Worry 7. What if my (divorced) mom or dad gets a new boyfriend/girl-friend?

Worry 8. What if that food I ate at school on Monday gives me food poisoning?

Worry 9. I might get a bad grade in chemistry.

Worry 10. My friends don't seem to like me anymore.

Worry 11. I think my grades in biology from last year aren't good enough to get me into my favorite college.

Worry 12. My friend has not responded to my text today. Does she still like me?

Worry 13. My history teacher seemed a little weird when we were talking today. Maybe I got a bad grade on that report.

Worry 14. My mom/dad has been working late a lot. I wonder if she/he will fall asleep while driving and get in a wreck.

Gameplay. The Character and Worry Cards are shuffled separately, and the signs are placed side by side in front of the players.

1. Player 1 draws a Character Card and reads the description.
2. Player 1 draws and reads a Worry Card.
3. Player 1 considers, thinking aloud, which of the four signs ("Worry Now," "Worry Later," "No Worry," "Not Sure") fits best for that Worry Card, considering the character described on the Character Card. Player 1 places the Worry Card on one of the signs and explains why he chose that sign.
4. The other player gives his/her opinion about the choice.
5. Player 1 repeats steps 2–4 for four Worry Cards, still using the first Character Card.
6. Then, Player 2 draws the next Character Card and play continues as described above.

Optional Bonus Round. Players sort through the Worry Cards in each resulting stack as follows:

• **Worry Now.** For these worries, the players take turns describing what the character could do to cope with the situation.

• **Worry Later.** For these worries, the players do two things. First, they talk about how they would "change the channel" on a worry like this, as they think it best to worry later. Second, they take turns telling *when* they think worrying about the concern would make sense. Another way to think about this is: What would need to happen to move this worry into the "Worry Now" pile? If the worries are broad ones, like, "What if I fail algebra?" the players could break the worry into smaller parts, like "How will I do on the next algebra assignment?" and "How will the next algebra test go?"

  • **Not Sure.** Using a "Not Sure" category can be tricky, and some therapists may want to consider not having one. Still, some clients who worry a lot are perfectionists and will worry excessively about choosing the right category for each worry in this game. For those clients, a "Not Sure" category can help move the game along. However, it is important to go back through the "Not Sure" group and engage in some Socratic questioning toward two different ends. First, some "Not Sure" worries can be recategorized after additional consideration. Second, it may be useful to have a broader conversation about the difficulty of categorizing worries. The therapist might ask, "What would happen if you did categorize these worries?" or "What would be the worst thing?" or "What if you categorized them wrong?" or "How would you know if you did it wrong?"

  When sorting through the "Not Sure" group for a second time, and after exploring the feared consequences, the therapist might also consider a gentle but forced-choice procedure. Here, the client is asked for his best guess for each worry (worry now, worry later, or no worry). It may be helpful to take anxiety ratings both before and after having the client make the choice, much like one does when conducting an exposure task, as the categorization may be considered an exposure for some clients. Forcing a choice not only helps the client learn the worry triage concept but also exposes the client to making a choice in the face of uncertainty. Once the choice has been made, the therapist can help the client to observe and note which of the feared consequences came to pass.

  • **No Worry.** For these worries, the players take one additional step, describing what possible changes would move the worry into the "Worry Later" or "Worry Now" category.

Step 4. Using Thoughts to Deal with Sadness

Overview

Cognitive interventions were first designed for application with depressed clients; however, there are challenges in using cognitive strategies with depressed clients for which adaptation may be helpful. One particular topic requiring some discussion is the challenge that has been called *depressive realism*, or what may be pithily called *tough circumstances*. The idea here is that some clients are depressed not only (or even mostly) due to overly distorted views, but instead due to some very real and very unfortunate circumstances. The science of depressive realism is a controversial one, and a full discussion is beyond the scope of this module (see Kistner, Balthazar, Risi, & David, 2001; Moore & Fresco, 2007). Hence, it may be easier for the purposes of this module to use the phrase *tough circumstances*, focusing on clients who are depressed in part because their circumstances are demonstrably difficult and upsetting.

Finding evidence for alternatives to sad thoughts can be difficult when working with clients in tough circumstances. As an example, consider 11-year-old Darnell, whose irritability and sadness are driven in part by his perception that his mother does not want to spend time with him and is always yelling at him. For Darnell, a common thought is, "Mom doesn't like me." Unfortunately, in Darnell's case, there was more evidence that his perception was accurate than not. Although many parents have ambivalent feelings about their children, most love their children enough to provide evidence to counter thoughts like this. However, many therapists have worked with families where such evidence is less abundant. In fact, most therapists can probably think of a few cases in which they had serious doubts about the love a parent had for a client. Even if therapists do not doubt the parent's love, there may be cases where they know that the parent's own mental health and/or substance use issues cloud his or her ability to parent and clearly demonstrate love and caring.

So what to do when the client is picking up on some level of unfortunate truth?

Teach

Address Tough Circumstances and Look for Counterevidence

What follows are six steps that can be useful for clients whose depression or sadness is rooted in part in living in tough circumstances. Although these steps do involve some teaching (e.g., generating alternative thoughts, identifying ways to cope), some of the work here is simply to validate the client's experience.

Work to Understand the Tough Circumstance. The goal here is both assessment (for the therapist) and exploration (for the client). The functional assessment process, as described in Chapter 4, can guide the assessment work. What one is aiming to understand better is where the *truth* is for the particular situation. For example, recall Darnell, described earlier. Assessment involved conversations with his mother. As it turned out, she did regularly yell at him, and even threatened at times to send him to Honduras to live with his father. She let the treatment team know that Darnell reminded her so much of her ex-husband, whom she hated, that she often had trouble seeing them as separate people. The team then gathered information from the mother about what she liked or appreciated about Darnell. That list started off small but grew over time. Given the lack of cognitive focus, further description of the assessment is omitted here. Needless to say, though, the goal of this assessment is to see to what extent the client's beliefs are supported by *actual* and *current* data.

Assessment involves the client, too. In Darnell's case, the team helped him to gather evidence about his belief that his mother did not want to spend time with him. To accomplish this, the team relied on the cognitive strategies described in Module 7, including emphases on the cognitive triangle, identification of thinking traps, and playing the Thought Detective game.

When Possible, Address the Reasons for the Tough Circumstance. With the assessment process completed, therapist and client can engage in problem solving to address some aspects of the tough circumstance. Strategies may include working directly with a caregiver or another adult in the client's life whom the client cannot directly influence. A few quick examples follow.

Case 1: Manny. Seventeen-year-old Manuel (Manny) had refused to go to school for more than 2 years. The school perceived his failure to attend as an issue stemming from delinquency and not from anxious and sad feelings. After the assessment yielded this finding, work initially involved meeting with the guidance counselor and principal to help them understand that Manny was truly anxious. At first, the school personnel resisted a flexible approach to gradually getting Manny back into school full-time. They insisted that they would need to expel him for failure to attend unless he attended full days immediately. As this was exactly the perception the client had, this was *not* an instance where cognitive work alone would suffice. The therapist persisted, though, in explaining the nature of the therapeutic work and how the client's feelings of depression and his fear of having panic attacks drove his school refusal. With this persistent approach, and with the buy-in from one teacher who had a history of panic attacks herself, the school did a complete 180 and worked collaboratively to help the client gradually re-enter school.

Case 2: Shadow. Twelve-year-old Shadow lived part-time with her mother and part-time with her father and his wife. She described her time with mother as scary and sad and said that she believed her mother hated her. Some of the specific behavior Shadow described fit the criteria for emotional abuse, and that information was reported to Child Protective Services. The therapist also learned that the mother had been diagnosed with borderline personality disorder. Here again, the therapist took steps that were not cognitive strategies at all. Specifically, she referred the mother for her own therapy, and she worked with the family to engage in safety planning so that Shadow would be safe even if the mother behaved erratically. In addition, she worked with Shadow to use some cognitive strategies to help her cope.

Both of these cases demonstrate that tough circumstances sometimes require more from a therapist than just helping the client view the situation from a different perspective. Actively addressing such circumstances, although not a cognitive strategy itself, can be part of a treatment plan that involves teaching and practicing cognitive emotion regulation by clarifying where such an approach can be helpful and where action more than thinking is needed.

Keep Looking for Counterevidence. Even in the face of verifiable tough circumstances, one can encourage clients to keep their eyes open for counterevidence. Keeping hope alive represents an important path to resilience in the face of tough circumstances, and one way to keep hope alive is to look for and *hoard* pieces of counterevidence. Darnell's case provides a good example of this. As noted, his mother did indeed have some unfortunate, strongly negative feelings about Darnell. However, the team also believed that she did love him. So the goal was to help Darnell work up the courage to ask his mother to spend time with him. One simple way to practice this was to ask her to play a game of Uno with him during a session. She reluctantly agreed and then clearly enjoyed herself during the game. Although she later suggested that finding time for games in her busy schedule would be impossible, she indicated that she'd had fun playing. The therapist then met with Darnell individually and helped him think through this new evidence about his mother. Together, they agreed that his belief that she did not want to spend time with him at all could be amended slightly.

It is important to be clear about the goal in looking for counterevidence. Therapists are encouraged to help clients maintain hope by looking for some good news, which can almost always be found even in very difficult situations. But the recommendation does not stand in all cases. Some beliefs are truly not distorted and may, in fact, be entirely reasonable. However, many therapists, the author included, have had cases where it was easy to lose sight of the young green shoots of good news amid the tall weeds of tough circumstances that many clients encounter. Remaining optimistic and ever vigilant for good news is a particularly useful stance to take as a therapist of clients in tough circumstances. That way, it will be easier to notice small changes in positive directions. That said, there are times when even the most optimistic therapists have to admit that a client's circumstance is just plain tough and unlikely to change. That is when the next two steps become important.

One Tough Circumstance Does Not Mean That Everything Is a Tough Circumstance. As noted, it can be easy in cases awash with tough circumstances to focus on the most intractable problems. Therapists do it because the big, hard-to-solve problems are like the 500-pound gorilla in the room. "How can I do any work with that beast in here?" one might ask. Clients do it because they have pushed and pulled on the gorilla for so long to no avail. A problem arises, though, when clients (and sometimes even therapists) overgeneralize from their experiences with the intractable problem. In doing so, both may overlook some circumstances that are not so tough and that can be coped with.

For example, consider a depressed 14-year-old client named Daphne who lives with her mother and her father. The father had only reappeared a few months earlier and was dying of cancer. Daphne's mother was so troubled by the father being around (they had divorced years earlier and he'd had very little contact with the family since) that she effectively moved out and went to live with her boyfriend, leaving Daphne to care for her dying father.

A temptation in this case was to focus on these very tough circumstances, on which there was surely work to be done. But in focusing on this troubling family dynamic, the treatment team at first overlooked other areas of Daphne's life over which she did have some control. For example, her school performance was declining because she was sad and feeling like her efforts would not matter. Once this issue was discovered, both cognitive work and problem solving were applied. She was willing to test her belief that nothing she did would matter and agreed to do her homework and study for tests. Working with therapist, she set up a schedule for completing her schoolwork. Together, she and her therapist tracked her school performance. Lo and behold, her efforts did yield dividends. The therapist helped Daphne to see the difference between her school circumstances, which were within her control, and some of her other circumstances, which were much less if at all within her control. In short, Daphne learned that although some things were out of her control, not all of them were.

For the Tough Circumstance(s) That Remain(s), Find Ways to Cope (and Maybe Give Them a Name).
Despite all best efforts, some tough circumstances will remain and the client will be challenged with accepting and coping with the truth of those circumstances. The goal here is to help clients acknowledge the problem as one that will not likely go away and identify ways to cope, some of which will involve cognitive strategies.

For the case of Shadow, described earlier, whose mother was ragingly mean to her at times, the therapist believed it was possible that the mother could eventually change her behavior. But the therapist also had to acknowledge that any change was not likely going to happen quickly; pretending that it would was not going to serve Shadow well. So the therapist validated Shadow's perceptions about her mother's behavior: sometimes she did indeed act in ways that were scary and upsetting. In a sense, the therapist was to confirming Shadow's perceptions. For Shadow, this was important because this was her mother, and rare is the person who sees her parents very clearly, and Shadow's mother was telling Shadow that she was not seeing things correctly. So from a cognitive perspective, confirming Shadow's perceptions of her mother helped her develop confidence in her perceptions in general.

Next, the goal was to help Shadow figure out how to cope when her mother was having trouble acting in an appropriately parental manner. Although the therapist engaged in a number of interventions relevant to this goal, one is particularly relevant to this chapter. Specifically, the therapist worked with Shadow to explore the possibility that her mother's behavior was not as personal as Shadow feared. That is, although Shadow's mother was indeed mean sometimes, the therapist and client worked to test Shadow's thought that the mother's meanness was Shadow's fault. They used the detective metaphor and gathered clues, some of which were tough to discuss. For example, Shadow noted that her mother was much meaner when she was drinking or when she forgot to take her medications. The therapist and Shadow began using the idea that Shadow's mother had a problem that sometimes led to her being unkind. Shadow decided to call this problem her mother's "broken leg." This cognitive strategy allowed Shadow to take a step back when her mother was acting irrationally and remind herself, "My mother's broken leg is acting up. It's not because of me. What she's saying now is because of her broken leg."

Practice: Activities and Games

There are no games or activities specific to the step related to dealing with sadness, although the Worry Sort game can be useful for clients who are sad, as worries and depression often co-occur. Furthermore, any of the three games from Module 7 are useful in dealing with sad feelings.

Step 5. Using Thoughts to Deal with Fears

Overview

Risk overestimation and catastrophization are common thinking patterns for fearful, anxious clients. Although many evidence-based treatments for anxiety in youth focus on exposure alone, other evidence-based approaches include cognitive techniques as one way to reduce anxiety and encourage approach behavior.

Teach

Know How the Body's Alarm System Works—and How It Makes Mistakes

A cornerstone of anxiety treatment from a cognitive-behavioral perspective is helping clients understand the difference between false and real alarms. *False alarms* occur when the body's sympathetic nervous system is activated but there is no true life-or-death danger. Instead, there is an exaggeration of threat (or overestimation of the chances a real threat will occur). Because the body does not know the difference between a real and false alarm, much like a car alarm does not know the difference between a car thief and a bump from another car, the feeling *inside* will suggest that the alarm is a real one. A goal of cognitive work is to help clients distinguish between these false and real alarms. In the case of false alarms, a therapist can proceed with cognitive work as described in Module 7.

Real alarms are situations in which the body has a fight-or-flight reaction and the reaction is warranted. That is, the situation is a real challenge to the survival or physical integrity of the client. A few examples: (1) encountering a bear on the trail; (2) a credible, severe physical threat from a peer; (3) abuse from a parent, caregiver, or adult; and (4) a sudden medical emergency befalling the client or someone the client knows (e.g., parent, sibling, friend). In these and other real-alarm situations, cognitive work aimed at correcting misperceptions is clearly not advisable. So what does one do? The following three steps represent one way.

Assess the Threat. The *real alarm–false alarm* dichotomy is misleading. There is plenty of gray area with regard to threat. First, some clients are going to be temperamentally more sensitive to threats. That is, one client's real alarm will be another client's false alarm. Second, therapists also have thresholds for what constitutes a real versus false alarm. When training therapists in our doctoral program, I have had many animated discussions about the threat involved in various situations clients raise in the course of therapy. For example, peers are not always friendly and accepting, but most peer situations are not real alarms, even if teasing becomes "nasty" and a client is in tears. On the other hand, armed peers or peers who credibly threaten harm or behave in a cruel fashion are more likely real alarms.

When conducting assessment of threat, the therapist should act as captain of the impartiality squad (see Module 7). A client's fear can exaggerate both the client and therapist's perception of threat. Furthermore, the use of certain buzzwords, like "bullied," or even a hysterical presentation of the client's problems by the client (or caregiver), can encourage the therapist to assign a higher level of threat than may be warranted. Snap judgments by therapists about threat levels are, like most snap judgments, prone to error. Snap judgments on the part of the therapist also model for clients and their caregivers a lack of careful consideration. If therapists assess well and thoroughly, they will be much better prepared to help the client cope optimally with whatever the stressor is.

A side note on stress is warranted here. It is important to remember that stress by itself is not dangerous, and avoiding stress should not be a primary life goal. Experience coping with stress is good preparation for those dealing with those stressors that will come later. And come they will! Research suggests that the best stressors, the ones that help us learn and grow, are both predictable and controllable. But even stressors that are *un*predictable and *un*controllable can be opportunities to improve our coping skills, thereby building self-efficacy and the confidence to face future difficulties.

This discussion on the benefits of stress is important because sometimes caregivers (and even therapists) approach children with an apparent belief that they should be shielded from stress and the resultant suffering. By no means is the recommendation here that adults should purposely add stress to children's lives. However, because stressful situations are inevitable, a very good way for children to learn that they can handle stressful situations (and almost all children can handle them) is for them to face those situations, ideally with some preparation, and with some discussion afterward as to how things went.

For False Alarms: Approach, Expose, and Do Some Cognitive Work. As noted already, if the threat assessment leads therapist and client to conclude that that the situation, while stressful, does not pose an actual danger, then cognitive work along with other strategies (e.g., skill building, exposure) may be appropriate.

For Actual Threats: Use a Combination of Safety Planning, Problem Solving, and Cognitive Coping. When learning about exposure therapy, therapists sometimes worry that exposure means exposing clients to danger. For example, they might ask, "What do I do if my client is afraid that his dad is going to hit him? His dad might actually hit him." Given that this is a real threat, suggesting the use of exposure therapy is, of course, clinically unethical. Exposure is the intervention of choice only for *false alarms*, when the client will not be in danger (and might even receive benefit) from confronting a stressor.

For real threats, the first steps are safety planning and problem solving, topics that are the domain of other books. Once some semblance of safety is established, there are three cognitive interventions that can be helpful for clients in these situations.

The first is an a priori strategy that could be thought of as the *safety plan reminder*. First, therapists must do a good job with safety planning and problem solving. With that work in hand, therapists can help the client remember all of the steps that have been taken to reduce the risks, using Socratic questions. Again, remember that fear leads the mind to exaggerate risks and overlook safeguards. Helping clients remember the steps they and others have taken to keep them safe or reduce risks can help to instill a small sense of control as well as focus them on the fact that they are being supported.

The final two cognitive interventions are both post hoc options and assume that a bad situation has occurred despite safety planning. The first is classic *make-lemonade-out-of-lemons* thinking. Sometimes there is not room, in the beginning or ever, for seeing the good aspect(s) of an event; however, something good can often be found even in difficult situations. For example, consider a client with an abusive parent or caregiver who has been put in prison. Although the adult did some terrible things, that person is now locked away and the client and other children are safe.

The second post hoc strategy could be called *resiliency thinking*. The goal here is to encourage the client to consider the fact that although the outcome was terrible, she coped with a challenging situation. It can be useful to have the client identify fictional or real-life people who also have faced struggles and coped with them bravely. The therapist might ask the client to describe those individuals and then build a set of descriptors that could be applied to the client herself. The following excerpt provides an example of this strategy. Liz is a 13-year-old whose real-alarm fear is that her mother will become very sick. Her mother has brain cancer and although there is aggressive treatment under way, the prognosis is not good. Here, the therapist and client talk some about the resilience of Harry Potter, the fictional teenager featured in the eponymous book series.

THERAPIST: What about Harry Potter? He had a ton of tough things happen to him.

LIZ: Yeah. Like losing his parents. And then losing his godfather. And then all the kids were mean to him that year, thinking he was crazy or something. And having Voldemort trying to kill him all the time.

THERAPIST: How would you describe Harry? Let's list some words that describe him.

LIZ: You mean like brave? Tough?

THERAPIST: Do you know the word *resilient?*

LIZ: Um, maybe. It means, um, I don't know.

THERAPIST: Resilient means that you handle tough things and bounce back.

LIZ: That definitely describes Harry.

THERAPIST: How about persistent? That means like . . .

LIZ: I know that one. It means you keep at something. Yeah, that's a good one for Harry.

THERAPIST: What if he thought he deserved the bad things that happened to him, like losing his parents and his godfather? Would you agree with him?

LIZ: No way.

THERAPIST: Okay, so our list has brave, tough, resilient, and persistent. Let's start there. How well do these words fit you?

LIZ: Brave? Not.

THERAPIST: Tell me why not.

LIZ: I'm not brave. I get super scared when bad things happen.

THERAPIST: Does brave mean you can't be afraid too? Was Harry Potter ever afraid?

At first, clients may resist positive labels. With patient consideration of the evidence, though, even they may find that the case for those labels becomes more and more compelling.

Resiliency thinking does not change a bad situation, of course, but it does help clients to place their real alarms in perspective and to reflect on their strengths and abilities to handle very different circumstances.

Practice: Activities and Games

There are no games or activities specific to the step related to dealing with fears. As with the section on sadness, the three games found in Module 7 are helpful ones for coping with fear thoughts and can be used to teach some of the points here.

References

Arnold, M. B., & Gasson, J. A. (1954). *The human person: An approach to an integral theory of personality*. Oxford, UK: Ronald Press.

Biederman, J., Rosenbaum, J. F., Bolduc-Murphy, E. A., Faraone, S. V., Chaloff, J., Hirshfeld, D. R., et al. (1993). Behavioral inhibition as a temperamental risk factor for anxiety disorders. *Child and Adolescent Psychiatric Clinics of North America, 2,* 667–684.

Calkins, S. D. (1994). Origins and outcomes of individual differences in emotion regulation. *Monographs of the Society for Research in Child Development, 59,* 53–72.

Calkins, S. D. (2007). The emergence of self-regulation: Biological and behavioral control mechanisms supporting toddler competencies. In C. A. Brownell & C. B. Kopp (Eds.), *Socioemotional development in the toddler years: Transitions and transformations* (pp. 261–284). New York: Guilford Press.

Calkins, S. D., & Fox, N. A. (2002). Self-regulatory processes in early personality development: A multilevel approach to the study of childhood social withdrawal and aggression. *Development and Psychopathology, 14,* 477–498.

Callaghan, P. (2004). Exercise: a neglected intervention in mental health care. *Journal of Psychiatric and Mental Health Nursing 11,* 476–483.

Campos, J. J., Campos, R. G., & Barrett, K. C. (1989). Emergent themes in the study of emotional development and emotion regulation. *Developmental Psychology, 25,* 394–402.

Campos, J. J., Frankel, C. B., & Camras, L. (2004). On the nature of emotion regulation. *Child Development, 75,* 377–394.

Camras, L. A., & Allison, K. (1985). Children's understanding of emotional facial expressions and verbal labels. *Journal of Nonverbal Behavior, 9,* 84–94.

Cassidy, J., Parke, R. D., Butkovsky, L., & Braungart, J. M. (1992). Family–peer connections: The roles of emotional expressiveness within the family and children's understanding of emotions. *Child Development, 63,* 603–618.

Chambless, D. L., Sanderson, W. C., Shoham, V., Johnson, S. B., Pope, K. S., Crits-Chrisotph, P., et al. (1996). An update on empirically validated therapies. *The Clinical Psychologist, 49,* 5–18.

Chorney D. B., Detweiler M. F., Morris T. L., & Kuhn B. R. (2008). The interplay of sleep disturbance, anxiety, and depression in children. *Journal of Pediatric Psychology, 33*, 339–348.

Chorpita, B. F. (2007). *Modular cognitive-behavioral therapy for childhood anxiety disorders.* New York: Guilford Press.

Chorpita, B. F., & Daleiden, E. L. (2009). Mapping evidence-based treatments for children and adolescents: Application of the distillation and matching model to 615 treatments from 322 randomized trials. *Journal of Consulting and Clinical Psychology, 77*, 566–579.

Chorpita, B. F., Daleiden, E. L., & Weisz, J. R. (2005). Identifying and selecting the common elements of evidence based interventions: A distillation and matching model. *Mental Health Services Research, 7*, 5–20.

Chorpita, B. F., & Southam-Gerow, M. A. (2006). Fears and anxieties. In E. J. Mash & R. A. Barkley (Eds.), *Treatment of childhood disorders* (3rd ed., pp. 271–335). New York: Guilford Press.

Chorpita, B. F., Taylor, A. A., Francis, S. E., Moffitt, C., & Austin, A. A. (2004). Efficacy of modular cognitive behavior therapy for childhood anxiety disorders. *Behavior Therapy, 35*, 263–287.

Chorpita, B. F., & Weisz, J. R. (2009). *MATCH-ADTC: Modular approach to therapy for children with anxiety, depression, trauma, or conduct problems.* Satellite Beach, FL: PracticeWise.

Cole, P. M. (1986). Children's spontaneous control of facial expression. *Child Development, 57*, 1309–1321.

Cole, P. M., Michel, M. K., & Teti, L. O. (1994). The development of emotion regulation and dysregulation: A clinical perspective. *Monographs of the Society for Research in Child Development, 59*, 73–283.

Cummings, E. M., Hennessy, K. D., Rabideau, G. J., & Cicchetti, D. (1994). Responses of physically abused boys to interadult anger involving their mothers. *Development and Psychopathology, 6*, 31–41.

Darwin, C. (1872). *The expression of the emotions in man and animals.* London: Murray.

Denham, S. A. (2006). Emotional competence: Implications for social functioning. In J. L. Luby (Ed.), *Handbook of preschool mental health: Development, disorders and treatment* (pp. 23–44). New York: Guilford Press.

Denham, S. A., Mason, T., & Couchoud, E. A. (1995). Scaffolding young children's prosocial responsiveness: Preschoolers' responses to adult sadness, anger, and pain. *International Journal of Behavioral Development, 18*, 489–504.

Derryberry, D., & Reed, M. A. (1994). Temperament and the self-organization of personality. *Development and Psychopathology, 6*, 653–676.

Efran, J. A., Lukens, M. D., & Lukens, R. J. (1990). *Language, structure, and change: Frameworks of meaning in psychotherapy.* New York: Norton.

Ehrenreich, J. T., Southam-Gerow, M. A., Hourigan, S. E., Wright, L. R., Pincus, D. B., & Weisz, J. R. (2011). Examining similarities and differences in characteristics of anxious and depressed youth in two different clinical contexts. *Administration and Policy in Mental Health and Mental Health Services Research, 38*, 398–411.

Eisenberg, N., Cumberland, A., & Spinrad, T. L. (1998). Parental socialization of emotion. *Psychological Inquiry, 9*, 241–273.

Eisenberg, N., Fabes, R. A., Guthrie, I. K., Murphy, B. C., Maszk, P., Holmgren, R., et al. (1996).

The relations of regulation and emotionality to problem behavior in elementary school children. *Development and Psychopathology, 8,* 141–162.

Eisenberg, N., Fabes, R. A., Shepard, S. A., Murphy, B. C., Guthrie, I. K., Jones, S., et al. (1997). Contemporaneous and longitudinal prediction of children's social functioning from regulation and emotionality. *Child Development, 68,* 647–664.

Eisenberg, N., & Lennon, R. (1983). Sex differences in empathy and related capacities. *Psychological Bulletin, 94,* 100–131.

Ekman, P. (1992). Are there basic emotions? *Psychological Review, 99,* 550–553.

Faber, A., & Mazlish, E. (1995). *How to talk so kids can learn at home and in school.* New York: Scribner.

Fiese, B. H., Foley, K., P. & Spagnola, M. (2006). Routine and ritual elements in family mealtimes: Contexts for child well-being and family identity. *New Directions in Child and Adolescent Development, 111,* 67–90.

Fox, K. (1999). The influence of physical activity on mental well-being. *Public Health Nutrition, 2,* 411–418.

Frattaroli, J. (2006). Experimental disclosure and its moderators: A meta-analysis. *Psychological Bulletin, 132,* 823–865.

Fredrickson, B. L. (1998). Cultivated emotions: Parental socialization of positive emotions and self-conscious emotions. *Psychological Inquiry, 9,* 279–281.

Freeman, K. A., & Miller, C. A. (2002). Behavioral case conceptualization for children and adolescents. In M. Hersen (Ed.), *Clinical behavior therapy: Adults and children* (pp. 239–255). New York: Wiley.

Friedberg, R. D., McClure, J. M., & Garcia, J. H. (2009). *Cognitive therapy techniques for children and adolescents: Tools for enhancing practice.* New York: Guilford Press.

Frijda, N. H. (1986). *The emotions.* New York: Cambridge University Press.

Ginott, H. (1965). *Between parent and child.* New York: Three Rivers Press.

Gottman, J. M., Katz, L. F., & Hooven, C. (1996). Parental meta-emotion philosophy and the emotional life of families: Theoretical models and preliminary data. *Journal of Family Psychology, 10,* 243–268.

Gray, J. A. (1990). Brain systems that mediate both emotion and cognition. *Cognition and Emotion, 4,* 269–288.

Greenberg, L. S. (2002) *Emotion-focused therapy: Coaching clients to work through feelings.* Washington, DC: American Psychological Association.

Greenberg, M. T., & Kusche, C. (2002). Executive summary. In D. S. Elliott (Series Ed.), *Blueprints for violence prevention: Promoting alternative thinking strategies* (pp. 7–18). Boulder: Institute of Behavioral Science, Regents of the University of Colorado.

Greenberg, M. T., Kusche, C. A., Cook, E. T., & Quamma, J. P. (1995). Promoting emotional competence in school-age children: The effects of the PATHS curriculum. *Development and Psychopathology, 7,* 117–136.

Gross, J. J., & Thompson, R. A. (2007). Emotion regulation: Conceptual foundations. In J. J. Gross (Ed.), *Handbook of emotion regulation* (pp. 3–24). New York: Guilford Press

Haley, J. (1991). *Problem-solving therapy* (2nd ed.). San Francisco: Jossey-Bass.

Haley, J. (1993). *Uncommon therapy.* New York: Norton.

Harvey A. G., Mullin B. C., & Hinshaw S. P. (2006). Sleep and circadian rhythms in children and adolescents with bipolar disorder. *Development and Psychopathology, 18,* 1147–1168.

Hayes, S. C., Strosahl, K. D., & Wilson, K. G. (1999). *Acceptance and commitment therapy: An experiential approach to behavior change.* New York: Guilford Press.

Henggeler, S. W., Schoenwald, S. K., Borduin, C. M., Rowland, M. D., & Cunningham, P. B. (2009). *Multisystemic therapy for antisocial behavior in children and adolescents* (2nd ed.). New York: Guilford Press.

Hofstede, G., Hofstede, G. J., & Minkov, M. (2010). *Cultures and organizations: Software of the mind* (3rd ed.). New York: McGraw-Hill.

Houlding, C., Schmidt, F., & Walker, D. (2010). Youth therapist strategies to enhance client homework completion. *Child and Adolescent Mental Health, 15,* 103–109.

Hughes, A. A., & Kendall, P. C. (2007). Prediction of cognitive behavior treatment outcome for children with anxiety disorders: Therapeutic relationship and homework compliance. *Behavioural and Cognitive Psychotherapy, 35,* 487–494.

Izard, C. (1977). *Human emotions.* New York: Plenum Press.

Izard, C. E., & Harris, P. (1995). Emotional development and developmental psychopathology. In D. Cicchetti & D. J. Cohen (Eds.), *Developmental psychopathology: Vol. 1. Theory and methods* (pp. 467–503). New York: Wiley.

Izard, C. E., Kagan, J., & Zajonc, R. B. (Eds.). (1984). *Emotions, cognition, and behavior.* New York: Cambridge University Press.

Jensen, A. L., & Weisz, J. R. (2002). Assessing match and mismatch between practitioner-generated and standardized interviewer-generated diagnoses for clinic-referred children and adolescents. *Journal of Consulting and Clinical Psychology, 70,* 158–168.

Kagan, J., Snidman, N., Arcus, D., & Reznick, J. S. (1994). *Galen's prophecy: Temperament in human nature.* New York: Basic Books.

Kendall, P. C. (Ed.). (2006). *Child and adolescent therapy: Cognitive-behavioral procedures* (3rd ed.). New York: Guilford Press.

Kendall, P. C., Hudson, J. L., Gosch, E., Flannery-Schroeder, E., & Suveg, C. (2008). Cognitive-behavioral therapy for anxiety disordered youth: A randomized clinical trial evaluating child and family modalities. *Journal of Consulting and Clinical Psychology, 76,* 282–297.

Kistner, J. A., Balthazor, M., Risi, S., & David, C. (2001). Adolescents' perceptions of peer acceptance: Is dysphoria associated with greater realism? *Journal of Social and Clinical Psychology, 20,* 69–84.

Kopp, C. B. (1989). Regulation of distress and negative emotions: A developmental view. *Developmental Psychology, 25,* 343–354.

Kovacs, M., Sherrill, J., George, C. J., Pollock, M., Tumuluru, R. V., & Ho, V. (2006). Contextual emotion-regulation therapy for childhood depression: Description and pilot testing of a new intervention. *Journal of the American Academy of Child & Adolescent Psychiatry, 45,* 892–903.

Kusché, C. A., Beilke, R. L., & Greenberg, M. T. (1988). *Kusche Affective Interview—Revised.* Unpublished manuscript, University of Washington, Seattle.

Larson, J., & Lochman, J. E. (2011). *Helping schoolchildren cope with anger: A cognitive-behavioral intervention* (2nd ed.). New York: Guilford Press.

Lazarus, R. S. (1991). Progress on a cognitive-motivational-relational theory of emotion. *American Psychologist, 46,* 819–834.

Lewis, M. (2008). Self-conscious emotions: Embarrassment, pride, shame, and guilt. In M. Lewis, J. M. Haviland-Jones, & L. F. Barrett (Eds.), *Handbook of emotions* (3rd ed., pp. 742–756). New York: Guilford Press.

Lewis, M., Haviland-Jones, J. M., & Barrett, L. F. (Eds.). (2008). *Handbook of emotions* (3rd ed.). New York: Guilford Press.

Linehan, M. M. (1993). *Cognitive-behavioral therapy of borderline personality disorder.* New York: Guilford Press.

Mash, E. J., & Barkley, R. A. (Eds.). (2007). *Assessment of childhood disorders.* New York: Guilford Press.

Masten, A. S., Burt, K. B., & Coatsworth, J. D. (2006). Competence and psychopathology. In D. Cicchetti & D. J. Cohen (Eds.), *Developmental psychopathology: Vol. 3. Risk, disorder, and adaptation* (2nd ed., pp. 696–738). Hoboken, NJ: Wiley.

Matsumoto, D. (2001). *Handbook of culture and psychology.* Oxford, UK: Oxford University Press.

Matsumoto, D., & Hwang, H. S. (2012). Culture and emotion: The integration of biological and cultural contributions. *Journal of Cross-Cultural Psychology, 43,* 91–118.

Mennin, D. S., & Farach, F. J. (2007). Emotion and evolving treatments for adult psychopathology. *Clinical Psychology: Science and Practice, 14,* 329–352.

Miklowitz, D. J., & Goldstein, T. R. (2010). Family-based approaches to treating bipolar disorder in adolescence: Family-focused therapy and dialectical behavior therapy. In D. J. Miklowitz & D. Cicchetti (Eds.), *Understanding bipolar disorder: A developmental psychopathology perspective* (pp. 466–493). New York: Guilford Press.

Miller, W. R., & Rollnick, S. (2013). *Motivational interviewing: Preparing people for change* (3rd ed.). New York: Guilford Press.

Mindell, J. A., Owens, J. A., & Carskadon, M. A. (1999). Developmental features of sleep. *Child and Adolescent Psychiatric Clinics of North America, 8,* 695–725.

Moore, M. T., & Fresco, D. M. (2007). Depressive realism and attributional style: Implications for individuals at risk for depression. *Behavior Therapy, 38,* 144–154.

Ortega, F. B., Ruiz, J. R., Castillo, M. J., & Sjöström, M. (2008). Physical fitness in childhood and adolescence: A powerful marker of health. *International Journal of Obesity, 32,* 1–11.

Paul, G. L. (1967). Outcome research in psychotherapy. *Journal of Consulting Psychology, 31,* 109–118.

Penza-Clyve, S., & Zeman, J. (2002). Initial validation of the Emotion Expression Scale for Children. *Journal of Clinical Child and Adolescent Psychology, 31,* 540–547.

Persons, J. B. (2008). *The case formulation approach to cognitive-behavior therapy.* New York: Guilford Press.

Reinecke, M., Dattilio, F., & Freeman, A. (2003). *Cognitive therapy with children and adolescents: A casebook for clinical practice* (2nd ed.). New York: Guilford Press.

Rueckert, L., & Naybar, N. (2008). Gender differences in empathy: The role of the right hemisphere. *Brain and Cognition, 67,* 162–167.

Saarni, C. (1984). An observational study of children's attempts to monitor their expressive behavior. *Child Development, 55,* 1504–1513.

Saarni, C. (1999). *The development of emotional competence.* New York: Guilford Press.

Schwartz, C. E., Snidman, N., & Kagan, J. (1996). Early childhood temperament as a determinant of externalizing behavior in adolescence. *Development and Psychopathology, 8,* 527–537.

Shields, A., & Cicchetti, D. (1997). Emotion regulation among school-age children: The development and validation of a new criterion Q-sort scale. *Developmental Psychology, 33,* 906–916.

Southam-Gerow, M. A., Chorpita, B. F., Miller, L. M., & Gleacher, A. A. (2008). Are children with anxiety disorders privately referred to a university clinic like those referred from the public mental health system? *Administration and Policy in Mental Health and Mental Health Services Research, 35*, 168–180.

Southam-Gerow, M. A., Hourigan, S. E., & Allin, R. B. (2009). Adapting evidence-based treatments for youth in partnership with mental health stakeholders. *Behavior Modification, 33*, 82–103.

Southam-Gerow, M. A., & Kendall, P. C. (2000). A preliminary study of the emotion understanding of youth referred for treatment of anxiety disorders. *Journal of Clinical Child Psychology, 29*, 319–327.

Southam-Gerow, M. A., Rodriguez, A., Chorpita, B. F., & Daleiden, E. (2012). Dissemination and implementation of evidence based treatments for youth: Challenges and recommendations. *Professional Psychology: Research and Practice.*

Southam-Gerow, M. A., Weisz, J. R., & Kendall, P. C. (2003). Youth with anxiety disorders in research and service clinics: Examining client differences and similarities. *Journal of Clinical Child and Adolescent Psychology, 32*, 375–385.

Stark, K. D., Sander, J., Hauser, M., Simpson, J., Schnoebelen, J., Glenn, R., et al. (2006). Depressive disorders during childhood and adolescence. In E. J. Mash & R. A. Barkley (Eds.), *Treatment of childhood disorders* (3rd ed., pp. 336–410). New York: Guilford Press.

Stathopoulou G., Powers M. B., Berry A. C., Smits J. A. J., & Otto M. W. (2006). Exercise interventions for mental health: A quantitative and qualitative review. *Clinical Psychology: Science and Practice, 13*, 179–193.

Stegge, H., & Terwogt, M. M. (2007). Awareness and regulation of emotion in typical and atypical development. In J. J. Gross (Ed.), *Handbook of emotion regulation* (pp. 269–286). New York: Guilford Press.

Suveg, C., Kendall, P. C., Comer, J., & Robin, J. A. (2006). A multiple-baseline evaluation of an emotion-focused cognitive-behavioral therapy for anxious youth. *Journal of Contemporary Psychotherapy, 36*, 77–85.

Suveg, C., Southam-Gerow, M., Goodman, K. L., & Kendall, P. C. (2007). The role of emotion theory and research in child therapy development. *Clinical Psychology: Science and Practice, 14*, 358–371.

Thompson, R. A. (1994). Emotion regulation: A theme in search of definition. *Monographs of the Society for Research in Child Development, 59*, 24–52.

Trentacosta, C. J., & Izard, C. E. (2007). Kindergarten children's emotion competence as a predictor of their academic competence in first grade. *Emotion, 7*, 77–88.

Triandis, H. C. (1995). *Individualism and collectivism.* Boulder, CO: Westview Press.

Underwood, M. K. (1997). Top ten pressing questions about the development of emotion regulation. *Motivation and Emotion, 21*, 127–146.

Weisz, J. R., Chorpita, B. F., Palinkas, L. A., Schoenwald, S. K., Miranda, J., Bearman, S. K., et al. (2012). Testing standard and modular designs for psychotherapy with youth depression, anxiety, and conduct problems: A randomized effectiveness trial. *Archives of General Psychiatry, 69*, 274–282.

Weisz, J. R., Southam-Gerow, M. A., Gordis, E. B., & Connor-Smith, J. K. (2003). Primary and secondary control enhancement training for youth depression: Applying the deployment-focused model of treatment development and testing. In A. E. Kazdin & J. R. Weisz (Eds.),

Evidence-based psychotherapies for children and adolescents (pp. 165–183). New York: Guilford Press.

Weisz, J. R., Suwanlert, S., Chaiyasit, W., & Walter, B. (1987). Over- and undercontrolled referral problems among children and adolescents from Thailand and the United States: The Wat and Wai of cultural differences. *Journal of Consulting and Clinical Psychology, 55,* 719–726.

Weisz, J. R., Suwanlert, S., Chaiyasit, W., Weiss, B., Achenbach, T., & Walter, B. (1987). Epidemiology of behavioral and emotional problems among Thai and American children: Parent reports for ages 6–11. *Journal of the American Academy of Child and Adolescent Psychiatry, 26,* 890–897.

Weisz, J. R., Suwanlert, S., Chaiyasit, W., Weiss, B., Walter, B., & Anderson, W. (1988). Thai and American perspectives on over- and undercontrolled child behavior problems: Exploring the threshold model among parents, teachers, and psychologists. *Journal of Consulting and Clinical Psychology, 56,* 601–609.

Werner, H. (1957). The concept of development from a comparative and organismic point of view. In D. Harris (Ed.), *The concept of development.* Minneapolis: University of Minnesota Press.

White, S. W. (2011). *Social skills training for children with Asperger syndrome and high-functioning autism.* New York: Guilford Press.

Wood, J. J., & McLeod, B. D. (2007). *Child anxiety disorders: A family-based treatment manual for practitioners.* New York: Norton.

Zeman J., & Shipman K. (1997). Social-contextual influences on expectancies for managing anger and sadness: The transition from middle childhood to adolescence. *Developmental Psychology, 33,* 917–924

Zeman, J., Shipman, K., & Suveg, C. (2002). Anger and sadness regulation: Predictions to internalizing and externalizing symptomatology in children. *Journal of Clinical Child and Adolescent Psychology, 31,* 393–398.

Index